BAJAN AFFAIR

By Pauline Pearce

'One million people commit suicide every year'
The World Health Organization

Pauline Pearce

All rights reserved, no part of this publication may be reproduced by any means, electronic, mechanical photocopying, documentary, film or in any other format without prior written permission of the publisher.

>Published by
>Chipmunkapublishing
>PO Box 6872
>Brentwood
>Essex CM13 1ZT
>United Kingdom

http://www.chipmunkapublishing.com

Copyright © Pauline Pearce 2007

Proof-read by Hannah Austin

BAJAN AFFAIR

Introduction

Allow me to introduce myself and give you a flavour of what is to follow. If you are of similar characteristic to me, these first few lines are of prime importance. These are the ones that determine whether the book is to be swiftly returned to the shelf or to become the next material for bedtime reading or holiday relaxation.

The authoress of the following is Pauline, a self-confessed 50-something eccentric, mother to Beth and wife of the long-suffering R—n (for the purposes of his anonymity/sanity/reputation, and in hope of preserving our twenty-five-year marriage, hereafter known as RT).

I have no shame in admitting to my eccentricity and, personally, find it adds colour and authenticity to each day of my life. Long live eccentricity. Long live humour save at no other's expense. It is this characteristic that has helped me on my personal journey from youth into something I describe as middle age – a period that filled me with initial dread until I learnt to adopt a different approach to the inevitable process of ageing.

I had originally thought that to die young in the full flush of youth (and, dare I say it, beauty) was far better than to watch face and body deteriorate in age. But now, faced with this reality, I appreciate there is so much more of life I desire to experience and have not yet had the opportunity to.

The mirror does not deceive though the mind oft can. I don't *feel* any older in my head but my facial features – not to mention the sagging boobs and bum and the hideous varicose veins – tell a different tale.

Growing older had never been of concern to me in my thirties or even forties but somehow, I went to bed on the 21st February 2006 a reasonably content 49-year-old and woke on the 22nd a discontented, quivering wreck – a 50 year old. As I gazed into the mirror, deep lines on my forehead and around my eyes seemed to have appeared as if by some voodoo curse. My lips appeared to have lost their original definition and shrunk in volume; chin and neck had merged into some vague area around shoulder level. Not a pretty sight to behold pre-early morning 'cuppa' at the dawning of a new decade!

Total despair. Total panic. Youth had left me in those eight hours I had slept.

I made an imminent decision. If I had to submit to the inevitable then my strategy would be to greet 'older' age with eccentricity – an endearing characteristic I had observed in others who were, in retrospect, perhaps a tad older than me. Better to begin early than not at all. I certainly did not want to turn into one of the notorious 'grumpy old women' portrayed on TV and with whom I had, more often than not, worked with in my role as psychotherapist.

It has been – once in mindset – something of a naturally occurring, even enjoyable evolution these past twelve months, assisted perhaps by the confidence that often comes to those of more senior years. After all, we've had a little more time than those luscious youngsters to try life out and discover a few more answers to its ever-posing questions.

A shift in life perception began and reactions to the unexpected events in which we inevitably get caught, both positive and negative.

This new era also marked the beginning of my literary career – something I had always wanted to pursue but never had the tenacity to apply myself to.

My first book, *Full Circle*, was published in 2006 after years of literal blood, sweat and tears. This was not so much in the penning of said script but in the monumental attempt to find a publisher who would take my (dare I say, without sounding pompous) literary talent seriously. Thanks go to Jason Pegler.

I digress; necessity requires me to return to this current rendition.

Bajan Affair tells of a holiday RT and I were

fortunate enough to spend on the Caribbean island of Barbados. It was written as a daily diary and hopefully coveys both a humour and, at times, pathos that I trust the reader will enjoy. It does not describe an affair of the heart with an individual but a seduction that comes from its inhabitants (almost without exception), their way of living and being. It also comes from the great beauty of the island and the anticipation with which I awoke each morning, for the adventure that day might – and inevitably did – bring.

I hope you will bear with me as I give explanation as to why we travelled to these far flung shores – a setting of the scene – as I draw this introduction to a close. The following becomes a little more serious but, believe me, there is light (and humour) at the end of this proverbial 'tunnel'.

The last few months of 2003 – certainly from October onwards – had been a difficult time for both RT and self.

I had been admitted to hospital with a suspected heart attack in the October. What I considered indigestion, RT interpreted as some form of problem with my heart. He phoned 999 and despite my protests I was soon being whisked away by ambulance to a coronary care unit!

I spent twelve days there. I attempted to discharge myself on several occasions but was told in no uncertain terms that it was unwise to until I had

BAJAN AFFAIR

some definite diagnosis, as there was a great possibility I could drop dead at any given moment. To disregard such advice would have been sure foolishness, so captive I remained.

The medics eventually ruled out the heart attack theory but then, in their wisdom, suggested the problem might be angina. After varying tests disproved this diagnosis, it mutated to *intermittent* angina, and an investigative angiogram was recommended.

To those unfamiliar with this terminology, allow me to explain. An angiogram is a procedure in which a wire is inserted into the groin and then – by some invasive procedure – 'threaded through' to the target area of the heart. Dye is injected into the artery and winds its merry way to this area, highlighting any defect or malfunction – all illuminated in brilliant Technicolor on a viewing screen. Hideous thought to one who faints at the mere prospect of a blood test.

The consent form for this procedure was terrifying, to say the least. There were possibilities of having a full-blown heart attack or stroke, or even losing a leg. I was extremely reluctant to sign and the young doctor who handed me the form admitted that he would not want to commit his signature to this either. I thought the whole idea was for the medic to give the anxious patient confidence in *any* investigative procedure, not to add to the neurosis. If this young man was a student, I do wonder how far he will progress in his medical career. As honest as he might have been (a characteristic I would usually admire) he most certainly did not possess a reassuring bedside manner.

Despite this I did eventually consent to the procedure, but only after demanding heavy-duty sedation. I knew the only way out of hospital was to prove that my original diagnosis (a digestive disorder) was the most likely scenario, but also wanted to ascertain that I wouldn't 'meet my Maker' shortly after stepping over the threshold of my home.

The procedure carried out, the results were immediately divulged – NO angina of any description present. This, after twelve days, finally allowed for discharge – but only on the condition that I would be attached to a heart monitor for twenty-four hours. Would they never give up on their attempt to find *something*?!

Might I add that, midway through my hospital admission, I had moved from standard NHS treatment into the realms of private medicine due to long-standing membership of an underused health scheme. It was all becoming, cynically, much clearer to me. Would the NHS provide so varied a range of investigations at such great expense? As an employee of the NHS, I thought it surely would not. But in the world of private medicine, the sky – and attendant cost – is, as they say, the limit.

Finally, the monitor un-strapped, the recording within decoded, a diagnostic proclamation was made by the eminent cardiologist that Pauline Pearce most definitely had not suffered, was not suffering, and in the immediate future looked most unlikely to suffer from any form of heart disease.

I was, finally and most definitely, discharged from any further coronary investigation/care with the knowledge that my heart was probably the healthiest organ in my entire body!

However, this entire episode had resulted in RT and me reassessing our lives in totality, even to the extent of how our income was spent. The phrase that reverberated in my head was 'life is not a dress rehearsal'. That is, we have but the one – as far as we humanly know – and have little idea what we will face as each day progresses, be this positive or negative.

We had always wanted to travel – to see more of this vast and wonderful world. Our new philosophy was 'topsy-turvy' thinking for the sensible middle-aged couple we had become – redecorating the house on a regular basis; replacing frayed carpeting and old furniture for new as finance allowed; saving perhaps more money (we were fortunate enough to be able to do this) than we needed for the 'rainy day' that, heaven forbid, may come. RT's employment seemed relatively secure

– twenty-five years' service in and ten years to retirement – and I had just become a second wage earner, after years of being mum-at-home. Our daughter had fled the nest post-university and was not financially dependent on us to the same degree. How about if my income became not merely 'practical' money to, for example, assist in renewing the car every three years, but instead was to become 'fun money'? Money to be spent on travelling – to visit those far flung shores that we had but dreamed of and had decided we would visit one day?

But what if 'one day' didn't come? I hadn't, after all, suffered a heart attack; it had been a false alarm. But what if the reality had been that it *had* been Pauline's time to meet her Maker, or if RT was to have a serious accident in the car and meet his?

In March 2003 I was fortunate enough to gain employment as a counsellor in a large primary care practice in north Liverpool. To earn money from my endeavours was an amazingly new experience, having worked in the voluntary sector for several years (not that I begrudge a single moment of this). To earn money in a profession that is my passion was an added bonus. This was the money RT and I decided was to take us to the glorious island of Barbados. Had it not been for my salary, a luxury such as this would have been but a dream. Hence, at reasonably short notice, the holiday was booked before any change of

BAJAN AFFAIR

mind came about. For once, impulsion took a lead and everyday practicalities were laid aside.

Sadly, in October 2003, RT's dad died. We spent many weeks going back and forth to North Yorkshire to be with his Mum, making funeral arrangements and afterwards assisting her with financial affairs. We were extremely tired and Christmas and New Year, a sad time for us without RT's Father, were especially difficult.

I hung on by my fingertips to get through the first two weeks of work in the New Year, knowing we had booked this most-needed holiday.

And then, the day arrived. We had not enjoyed its anticipation as we should and had feelings of guilt following our problems in the UK. But out to Barbados we flew, and so began the Bajan Affair.

What follows is the unabridged diary of Pauline Pearce in her tropical paradise. In the first few days I had little idea of the potential of my scribblings, let alone that I might attempt to publish my work. Initially, the diary was a little sketchy, having been written retrospectively. However, it soon became a detailed account, written ritualistically every evening, in an attempt to avoid losing the essence of those hours. From something quite small a monster grew!

I hope you enjoy reading it as much as I enjoyed putting pen to paper at the close of each magical day.

BAJAN AFFAIR

PROLOGUE:

Sunset Over Barbados

How can words do justice to one of the most beautiful sights on the island of Barbados, as the sun sets on the western horizon?

As I sit and watch the ruby-red sun sinking into the calm Waters of the Caribbean I drink in an intoxicating experience – more potent than the finest wine or vintage champagne; more addictive each time I view and live this experience; more seductive than a lovers caress.

How can I describe the perfection of this picture? How can I convey its beauty? Words seem insignificant.

If I were an artist with colours and textures at hand, could I even then catch this beauty on canvas?

Sunset of God's creation, you cannot be contained or tamed as a wild animal confined. You live; you breathe; you have life eternal; your vibrant colour changes with each passing moment of majesty.

Each night I watch you. Each night you are a little different, but of no less magnificence. How amazing are your colours – the sky alight with fire of blazing red, fading slowly to shades of magenta, then pink.

The clouds, too, accentuate your beauty. Some nights they are as candyfloss but of the purest white; other nights clouds tinged with grey through which your light shines, casting shadows on the darkening blue of the sea, unique in their pattern and formation. Each night, you tell a differing story of light, shade and reflection on the water.

As hard as I try, my camera cannot depict your magnificence – so many photos taken, so many disappointments. Is it God, in his highest authority, saying to me: 'this is my creation, in all its glory. You are privileged to view my work through the eye of humanity. You cannot take it away in artificial form, be it on film or on canvas'?

Yet, his message falls on deaf ears. I strive for that perfect pictorial imagery. Time upon time, I fail.

In a blink of an eye, the sunset reaches its crescendo, only to wane and die. Darkness ensues but, even within this, there is a sweetness of its own. The stars soon display their own unique glory as they illuminate the evening sky. They tease and encourage the moon to join them.

As from time eternal, there comes a reassurance: day will surely follow night.

This is nature in its purest and unrefined form. With little doubt, such beauty comes from our

BAJAN AFFAIR

Creator, God. How could it be any less than this?

Pauline Pearce

Diary of my Bajan Affair

Monday, 19th January 2004

We left home at a civilised time in the morning, not in the dreaded early hours as had been the case on other occasions, necessitating the setting of three independent alarms for 4am in case two fail and you oversleep. The scenario then is that you usually cannot get to sleep until 2am and are enjoying a wonderfully relaxing slumber when the alarms jolt you awake, seemingly moments later.

We enjoyed an uneventful taxi journey to the airport, an uneventful check-in and an uneventful departure, only minutes later than displayed on the flight information board. Remember, reader, we were still in the domain of the civilised and sensible 'stiff upper lipped' UK.

I had felt rather annoyed beforehand. RT had been straining to close my suitcase and then weigh it. He declared the weight was well above the baggage allowance for the flight. Why are men so self-limiting when they pack? Why do we women need so many more essentials? Why do men – well, my man at least – have so little sympathy for our plight? I had packed all the heavy shoes, beach towels and copious bottles of pre-sun, during-sun and post-sun lotions into his case, hence he could not help me in my dilemma. I must have spent half an hour deciding what to take and what to leave – a stressful part of the day

BAJAN AFFAIR

as the taxi was due any minute! My case had been beautifully and carefully packed. Now it looked as if Customs had been rummaging through it, trying to find illicit contraband. Eventually, the decision was made. It had to be. The taxi was hooting outside the house and RT was in a rage, face turning redder by the minute. However, when checking in at Manchester Airport, RT realised he had been mistaken and we did have a greater baggage allowance than he had perceived. Was that a man in trouble?

We boarded the aircraft on time, but not before donning flight socks and self-medicating with copious amounts of aspirin to prevent DVT. I am not sure whether I should have swallowed the latter because I have had an ulcer in the past! The question was, what might cause the most potentially harmful damage? DVT was my decision and, as I had neither DVT nor internal bleeding either during or post-flight, I feel I made the correct decision.

The in-flight food was, as usual, fairly disgusting. The space for legs and wriggling about performing anti-DVT exercises was limited. In all, not a very comfortable passage of eight hours, yet the cabin crew were reasonably civil. Remember, this was a chartered and not a scheduled flight ('pack the devils in and make more money!').

The only anxiety on disembarking at Barbados was that we went off in a minibus leaving our luggage on the pavement. Would we be reunited at our hotel?

The system actually worked extremely well. The hotel (the Tropical Escape) was fine but a little shabby. How the holiday brochures lie! How they add intensity of colour or shoot scenes with a wide lens to add to their size or quality! This applied to certain parts of our hotel – the bedrooms, bar area and especially the minute swimming pool. But, let's face it, when you have a Caribbean beach minutes from the hotel, does that really matter?

We knew the hotel was not set on the beach and that there was a road between the accommodation and sea front, but we had not anticipated just how busy and noisy this road would be. Feelings of disappointed set in until we visited the incredible beach, just as the brochure had portrayed; no picture editing or distortion here. Another bonus was that our hotel had an area of free sun beds for residents and we could access unlimited icy drinks to cool us in the hot Bajan sunshine.

The Bajans employed at the hotel were extremely friendly and helpful; the food was copious and of good quality and the alcohol ran freely. I do not imbibe in the 'devil's juice' but there was also no lack of tea, coffee, non-alcoholic drinks and delicious fruit cocktails.

Our feelings towards the hotel were becoming

BAJAN AFFAIR

much more upbeat, to the extent that we were less aware of the traffic noise or annoyed at having been misled pictorially by the brochure. We were both tired after our long day and went to bed early that night. Adventure for real would begin the next morning.

Pauline Pearce

<u>Tuesday 20th January – Saturday 24th January</u>

I did explain that my narrative of the first few days is reasonably brief as it was written retrospectively. Here begins a general synopsis of Tuesday to Saturday:

1. Our holiday rep, Solange, was both helpful and unobtrusive and her local knowledge could not be criticised in any way.

2. We were beginning to really love the hotel and its little idiosyncrasies. For example, although the restaurant was enclosed on three sides with lovely ceiling fans to keep us cool, the fourth side, facing towards road, was open. This meant it was accessible to the birds. Some were gentle sparrow-like creatures, others not so charming miniatures of the UK blackbird - jet black with piercing yellow eyes. The former birds were quite timid but the black birds (you had to admire their audacity) would sit on nearby tables watching you eat, ready to pounce as you left your seat. The scenario was reminiscent of Alfred Hitchcock's classic movie *The Birds*. Needless to say, RT and I never left the table together to 'attack' the buffet. One of us always remained on guard once we had begun eating. On one occasion, a little black thief even had the audacity to land on the hot buffet food containers and peck at the contents. Suprisingly, neither of us suffered from any form of food poisoning nor other digestive disorder during our time in residence.

BAJAN AFFAIR

3. I discovered an amazing non-alcoholic cocktail at the hotel made by one particular barman. This involved a whole banana, a range of different fruit juices and copious amounts of ice, all whizzed together in a blender. It had the consistency of Complan (which I detest) but certainly did not taste like it. It was totally delicious yet I fear impossible to duplicate on our return to the UK. As for calories – probably as many as a female should consume in a whole day!

4. I wrote the dreaded postcards to relatives in the first few days. I always detest writing these and feel I cannot relax until they are completed and posted – duty; drudgery; Monday 6am alarm feelings. Why do I feel like this? Why can't I delight in sharing my holiday anecdotes with those who remain in the depths of a UK winter? Am I slothful, lazy or, on a more positive note, perhaps just too nice a person to want to make others envious of my vastly more idyllic location? Personally, I think it's just that I can't be bothered!

5. We visited a polo match (horses are my greatest passion) and sat by a white Bajan trainer of the equestrian strain. I learned all the ins and outs of the game and how the scoring system works. I came away (with bored husband in tow) a lot more knowledgeable and really enjoyed the experience. However, I did not like the fact that the polo players were all white, whilst the grooms were predominantly black. It was the first time on

the island that I had seen this type of division. White and black had seemed to rub shoulders in colourless equality. I was left with somewhat of a bad taste in my mouth.

This, in a nutshell, is the summary of the first few days. RT and I had been so tired after our extremely stressful few months that we did little more than sunbathe, eat, drink and sleep. Sheer bliss!

I'm sure to expand on the former would do little to engage your attention and only, in all probability, bore you. How many times can one describe a swim in the warmth of the iridescent Caribbean sea; the ritualistic daily sunbathing on the palm fringed beach; the over consumption of good food and drink, and the sheer delight of wakening to the never-disappointing Bajan sunshine? All simple pleasures, I'm certain you'll agree.

Now follows the 'meat and bones' part of my diary. I hope I am able to do justice in my chosen words to describe this small corner (island in all reality) of paradise nestling in the majestic Caribbean waters.

BAJAN AFFAIR

Sunday, 25th January

This was to be our first visit to Paynes Bay Pentecostal Church, and what an experience (forgive me if I become a little more serious for a while.)

We do attend an Evangelical church in the UK so perhaps we could be classed as 'happy clappy' worshippers – much as I hate that description. I would prefer to call it 'free worship'. We do not chant from a ritualistic prayer book and our services have more of a 'fluid' feel, definitely biblically based but more in touch with the 'here and now'; the everyday trials and issues we all face.

Paynes Bay church was definitely in the latter category and within these four walls I felt an abundant blessing from the Holy Spirit. Our two visits gave me so much during our time in Barbados, lifting me from lethargic spirituality to a place where I could recharge my spiritual batteries. I came, again, to feel purpose and God working in my life in a very real way.

In true Bajan style, the minister arrived for a 10am service at 10.15, driving a battered old mini-van crowded with members of his congregation.

We were welcomed with beaming smiles, hearty handshakes and even crushing bear hugs. The wonderful fact of being a Christian is that no matter where we may live or whatever colour our skin may be, we are all of God's family. To me, that is a powerful acknowledgement and the exact sense experienced in the Pentecostal church that very morning.

Christ's love shone out and was reflected within the service. I felt a real warmth – nothing to do with the blazing sun outside the church but a warmth within my heart that connected me to the congregation and service and reconnected me to the Lord.

Within the service, some of the Sunday school pupils (including adults) had been set a task to memorise verses from the King James Bible. They came up, one by one, and attempted to recite these before the congregation – a daunting task whether six years old or sixty! Some pupils were word-perfect whilst others needed some minor prompting. I could feel the congregation urging them to recount the verses and even filling in faltering or missing words. The applause after each individual finished his or her recitation was 'ear shattering'.

The joy and love the congregation had for the Lord shone from their happy, smiling faces. It washed away all inhibition as they praised, both in song and in word. There was a prayer time at one particular point; whilst gospel music played in the background - the minister's wife bowed a slightly

BAJAN AFFAIR

off-key cello, her daughter played the piano and a young black man kept time on drums Each person vocalised their own individual prayer, yet these in totality seemed to blend together in perfect spoken harmony.

Who could fail to be anything less than spirit-filled in that building and with that congregation of such great faith? Materially they had so little, yet spiritually they had riches beyond belief. I had entered that building with a heavy heart after recent circumstances. I left the same building a different person – strengthened in my faith and ready to take on whatever obstacles life might put before me. What an amazing two hours. Indeed, what a highlight to our whole Bajan experience.

After returning to the hotel for lunch, we packed our beach paraphernalia and set off towards the luminous turquoise sea. Even though the hotel was situated on a busy main road and there was no official pedestrian crossing, the politeness of the drivers amazed me. There could be a continuous stream of traffic from both directions and yet, once noticed, drivers from either side would stop and motion you across. There were no hooting horns or angry remarks from fellow motorists but a unified courtesy from all. Would this happen in the UK? I fear not.

On reaching the beach and selecting sun beds positioned as close as possible to the ice-cold drink provision, I began my ritualistic sunbathing whilst RT, fully clothed and hat bedecked ensured he had maximum sun protection and shade. Why do most northern Europeans have an obsession to turn pale skin into something dark and prune like? We know the sun is harmful and that not only do we run the risk of acquiring cancer, but also of prematurely ageing our skin. The sun, in its great strength, will further define wrinkles and age spots, as it sucks the moisture from outer defensive layers. Yet, the fact that our skin does change to a darker shade (despite perhaps burning and peeling during the process) makes us <u>feel</u> healthier and in general, happier. Often in the relaxing heat of the sun (or even sun bed) all sense leaves us and insanity invades. Soon, I will be returning to a cold, bleak February in the UK. No one, save myself, will see my potentially superb tan as I wrap myself in extra layers to keep the winter chills out. Pure madness, in retrospect, but perfect sanity in the moment!

After a relaxing afternoon on the beach, sunbathing interspersed with the occasional swim (as a relief from the heat of the sun) we returned to the hotel. The evening meal was, as usual, delicious and this 'all-inclusive' holiday package is definitely the reason for my rapidly expanding waistline. My weakness, unfortunately, is puddings. It has been known for me to return to the buffet several times for top-up desserts. Also, this being a priority, if I spot something totally tempting, I might even select my dessert/s pre starters or main course, to prevent particular

BAJAN AFFAIR

delights disappearing from the buffet and, horror upon horror, not being replaced! I feel ashamed to admit to such gluttony but I am an honest, if greedy, person!

We retired to bed a little earlier than usual, as the following morning we were to begin a new adventure. Our hire car was arriving and we planned an early start. What was to unfold with the Pearce's 'flying solo'? The dawning day would reveal all.

Pauline Pearce

<u>Monday, 26th January</u>

The much awaited day of freedom to roam the island on four wheels arrived and with it the anticipation of seeing 'raw' Barbados away from the main tourist areas. When booking the car and looking for the least expensive option we were filled with amazement that convertibles were, indeed, better value. Having hired cars in European destinations such as Greece, Italy and Spain, such conveyances are 'top of the range' – that is, far too expensive for people of modest income like ourselves.

The car arrived at the hotel an hour later than we had been told to expect it. However, for the more fluid Bajan timescale, this was not unreasonable. We had chosen a mini-moke with optional top covering but completely open-sided. By this I must explain there were no doors, merely a twelve-inch ledge to climb over, both at the front and rear. With my questionable balance it was quite a feat initially, getting in and out. However, as the day progressed brain and motor coordination improved and I became quite an expert at hopping in and out. The only reason we did not dispense with the top completely was due to RT's bald patch and fair, freckly skin. He is the only person I have ever seen sitting on the beach under a sun umbrella in peaked cap, dressed in t-shirt to the neck, shorts to knee, socks from knee to ankle and totally smothered in factor 40, yet still ending up with barbecued red skin.

BAJAN AFFAIR

Regarding the rental price, the fact that there were two holes positioned beneath both driver and passenger seats should have made alarm bells ring immediately. We were soon to discover their function.

At 10am we were experiencing wonderfully sunny weather conditions – brilliant blue skies with a mere smattering of white, billowing cloud. By 11am the cloud had increased and turned to a soft shade of grey and by 11.15 this had mutated into shades of deep charcoal verging on the blackest of granite.

Minutes later, we were caught in the midst of a tropical rainstorm. Rain with unimaginable ferocity swept through one side of the car to the other. The mini-moke, you may recall, had no doors and its occupants were fast soaking up the downpour. We took cover on a tree-lined side of the road in an attempt to evade the horizontal course of rain. I was, by now, reasonably well protected from the driving rain whereas the long-suffering RT was still getting drenched from the spray of passing cars (more expensive, fully watertight saloon hire cars, might I add). Eventually the rain eased and it was payback time for the reasonably dry passenger. As we turned a sharp bend the water which had collected on the roof of the car deluged off onto my seat and clothing.

However, as quickly as the rainstorm arrived, the

brilliant Bajan sun reappeared and, the car interior and occupants began to dry out. Within an hour, dripping hair and soggy shorts were but a memory.

It might seem impossible to lose one's direction on an island only twenty-one miles long and fourteen miles in diameter, but happen this did. It was mainly due to the navigator (myself) being totally bereft of a sense of direction and having something akin to dyslexia when confronted with a road map. Unfortunately, RT had lost his reading glasses in the car. They had literally been eaten up as we bumped along a road of many potholes. RT had rested them on a ventilation duct, which we later discovered had no grill. As the car jolted along, this resulted in the glasses being dropped into some subterranean cavity within the car interior. Despite frantic efforts to release the bonnet, it remained implacably in situ as if superglued.

One enraged husband was developing a remarkable resemblance to the fictional Victor Meldrew! The concern I have is that Victor is a figment of an author's imagination whereas my own dear 'Victor' is decidedly non-fictional flesh and blood! It is too surreal to believe that the author had somehow transcended time boundaries, had met with and studied RT and on his observation based this 'I don't believe it!' character. In all honesty, this person does exist in the embodiment of a very real individual.

BAJAN AFFAIR

Allow me to divert a little from our day of exploration to return to events of the previous day.

An example of <u>my</u> Victor's characteristics were that he had been thrown into paralytic anxiety on hearing reports, on the BBC World News, that north west England was entering a period of arctic weather with temperatures dropping to minus seven and below. In total panic, he immediately headed to the nearest Internet café (yes, even in paradise they exist!) and emailed a neighbour holding our house key. With ferocity of speed and two-fingered typing, he asked for the temperature of our central heating thermostat to be raised to prevent risk of burst pipes or whatever else might flood, damage or destroy our property.

The email response relieved RT greatly. Temperatures were apparently mild and yes, of course, if the arctic weather arrived, our neighbour would do as bidden. One anxiety removed for RT, but no doubt another would take its place – such is the usual pattern.

My sentiments on the house flooding scenario were that a) we are covered by insurance, and b) it would be an opportunity to replace frayed old carpets and MFI furniture (much of it now held together with superglue) for something maybe a little more upmarket. My comments were not appreciated!

Pauline Pearce

Away from the prospect of a Cheshire Ice Age, we return to a more pleasant agenda, if RT can keep the 'worry warts' at bay.

We eventually spent a glorious day exploring the east coast of the island, still losing our way at times, but getting lost in the warm sunshine with little agenda was quite acceptable. Back in the UK too many everyday deadlines have to be met. To have this day in aimless pursuit of simple pleasure felt quite perfect. Even in losing our way, there were unique scenarios for us to experience.

Driving in Barbados is an adventure in itself. The hire companies provide maps of the island but, as previously mentioned, when Pauline navigates, some roads disappear entirely whilst others emerge as if from nowhere.

Could the fault lie with the ordinance surveyor or does the problem originate from self? I imagine the latter. A simple change of direction, whether in the UK or Barbados, leaves me disorientated and RT fuming, if he has the misfortune to be driving.

However, in Barbados, losing bearings can actually be a pleasantly, positive experience.

At one point today, we were supposedly heading for an inland vantage point and, instead, found ourselves on a most wonderful beach, on the opposite side of the island. We sat on the shore, eating our (by now) lukewarm packed lunch whilst

BAJAN AFFAIR

drinking in the beautiful sight and sound of the Atlantic Ocean crashing over nearby rocks – majestic, white, foaming waves similar in appearance to freshly whipped cream.

The getting lost scenario (or, to use RT's now-more-chilled-out expression, 'we're not lost, merely temporarily unsure of where we are') had even brought something more positive to the situation. We had chance conversations with local characters whom we would not have had the opportunity to meet if we had been correctly en route.

Whenever we had stopped the car to consult the map, even for the shortest of time, no less than three individuals had attempted to come to our rescue.

The first was a cheerful elderly man astride pushbike; the second a jeep with darkened windows, pulling alongside us at a T-junction in a remote part of the island.

Re the latter incidence, my immediate reaction was ensuing panic, fearing a possible mugging or hijack. However, our faith was restored as the driver's window wound down revealing a polite young man pointing us in the direction we requested – another knight in shining armour to our rescue.

Pauline Pearce

Our final guides were in the form of eight Bajan soldiers, armed with rifles and seated in an open-backed army jeep – again, an initial wrongly perceived threat. I thought, perhaps, we'd strayed onto military territory and were being brought to task for so doing. Despite their lethal weapons, smiles spread across their handsome faces, displaying an inward beauty of character and soul. It felt more of a meeting with the 'lads' brigade' than with a mean and ferocious fighting force and defenders of the island. I do not say that in any terms of mockery but, again, just to stress the nature of these warm-hearted people.

On at least one of these occasions we had merely paused to take stock of our bearings and were most definitely not lost, despite navigator's incompetence. Yet, how could we refuse such generosity of spirit by admitting this?

Even if, as a tourist in Barbados, you may be driving in a quiet area, lost with no one in sight to guide or advise, I guarantee you will always arrive at a location perhaps even more special than the original planned destination.

We never quite reached anywhere today. Well, that's not quite the truth. We found Bathsheba – a little town on the eastern Atlantic coast, very different from the western side where we were based. The waves raged against the rocks in a most dramatic fashion. There the sea was to be admired for its strength and power but not, as in

BAJAN AFFAIR

the calm pastel shades of the west, to swim in.

Tomorrow would be our second and final day of four wheel exploration and perhaps we would reach the destinations we had planned for today but despite this, our experiences had been made fresh and memorable in many ways and as the Bajans sing in their reggae words, 'Don't worry. Keep happy. Everything's gonna be all right'.

I did believe this as I prepared for bed. Plans are of value but sometimes we become too rigid in trying to keep to them. If we could just adopt some of the Bajan attitude and our lives could be more fluid, would we be happier and more content? Some of our best experiences merely happen unplanned and occur out of the blue, and we would miss these if we let rigidity, rather than fluidity, rule our lives. Tomorrow will bring fresh experiences. We do not know what life has in store for us. Life is an adventure to be taken at leisure. It is certainly not a race.

Tuesday, 27th January

Having my morning wash today, I realised most of my fake tan had disappeared (washed off by the sea and copious showers) and now I was just as pale – if not paler – than when we first arrived. All educative advice about skin cancer and wrinkles quickly faded from memory as thoughts turned to abandoning the application of high factor sunscreen. Reasoning that possibly only my face would be visible to work colleagues on my return to the miseries of the UK winter, I decided this part of my anatomy would receive greater UV exposure. Up until then, I had been showing this part of my body great respect – expensive facial moisturiser (not my usual Superdrug economy special) with factor 50 sunscreen.

In the mirror this morning, the face reflecting back was that of a pallid Michael Jackson, with additional black bags under my eyes accentuating the whiteness of my skin.

Today, the original rumination of: 'I must protect my face at all costs to prevent skin dehydration with ensuing lines and wrinkles' gave way to: 'it's too late already. The lines, the wrinkles and crows' feet are already well established. Why not go, all out, for a tan? At least then, the bags under eyes will be less noticeable and I might even return to work looking slightly healthier than when I left!'

BAJAN AFFAIR

Accordingly, only one thin application of suncream was applied and my sunhat was abandoned. I will possibly regret this attitude when I am in my sixties with prune-like, paper-thin facial skin. However, if I were to be knocked over by a bus next week, I would, at least, die looking tanned and healthy (can a corpse look healthy?!) rather than pale and sickly when family and friends came to bid me farewell at the funeral directors'.

Today the sun was shining and the conditions for the mini-moke were perfect. I had my usual poolside visit before we left to see which local craftsmen had stalls set up, in my endeavour to find gifts for relatives back home. (It was the practice of the hotel to allow a small number of local craftsmen to display their ware in this manner each morning).

I found the ideal gift for Beth: a multi-coloured Rastafarian hat. She is, at present, 'into' hats (beanies) in a big way and this headgear would hopefully fit the image she'd latterly adopted. If it did not appeal, I could most certainly give it to my mum as a tea cosy. At eighty-eight years old, I was sure she would not recognise it for its intended purpose.

As we drove from the hotel, I felt a real excitement. We could now go to the wildlife sanctuary, which had been yesterday's plan, thwarted by us arriving as it was about to close after many hours spent confused and lost on winding roads and tracks en route to heaven-knows-where.

I, being the perfectly organised partner in the relationship, had packed my bag last night; it now contained sun cream; sunhat; my usual glasses; three extra pairs (one distance, one reading and one non-prescription sun shades) in case of loss or damage to the originals; all-important map; beach towels; daily medication; novel; guide book; short sleeved tee shirt in case of burnt shoulders; sleeveless tee shirt in case shoulders were OK and back was burnt; one pair of dry bikini bottoms (cannot bear wet bottom enveloped in dry shorts); antiseptic cream; midge repellent; plasters, and so on. You might now appreciate that this was an extremely large, bottomless bag that 'ate up' contents so completely that an eternity could be spent looking for one item, with no guarantee of its eventual retrieval.

RT only had to bring self and camera. He managed to bring himself but not the camera. I personally felt suicidal when this was discovered three-quarters of the way to the wildlife sanctuary. RT would not return to the hotel, being too impatient to get on with the day or, perhaps, too afraid we might get lost on the return journey, as we had done the day before.

I tried desperately to bring my Christian virtues to the fore and not let this develop into an argument

BAJAN AFFAIR

that would mar the whole day. I remained tight-lipped and silent (unusual for me) but **I** knew that **he** knew I was mad!

The animal reserve was amazing. There was an incredible array of differing and colourful species of animals, reptiles and birds, some known and present in the UK (if only in the zoo), others native to the island.

Where do I begin? Multi-coloured parrots; crimson flamingo; slowly ambling tortoises; prehistoric-like iguanas and armadillos; glorious fantailed peacocks; large black-billed toucans; mongoose; agouti (a cross between hare and guinea pig); caiman (alligator-like reptile); tiny native deer . . . the list continues. They mainly roamed free in the sanctuary, although certain species (of the winged variety) were in aviaries. So many potential photo opportunities, but no camera.

I internalised my anger. Maybe the Bajan attitude to life has affected me! I forcibly practised Christian thoughts of forgiveness and charity whilst fighting a raging battle of anger within. I remained very quiet for fear of opening my mouth and torrents of abuse issuing forth. I felt quite proud of my restraint.

As we left the reserve, I spotted a sign indicating that if you had not seen the green monkeys (the main attraction) you could have your ticket re-stamped and return, within two weeks, at no additional charge. I felt overjoyed. We could return another day (it was suggested between 3pm and 4pm – feeding time) and 'snap away', building up a pictorial memory of our visit. Waves of childlike joy and re-emerging love for husband engulfed me. Perhaps all was not lost.

It felt safe to speak and point this out to RT. However, his response was that he had already noticed this sign when we first arrived. Yet, he had not informed me! This was when Vesuvius erupted within me. Why had he not told me before? Christian charitable thoughts completely dispersed and RT became prey to a torrent of abuse, made all the greater by its suppression for the past hour and a half!

To move on swiftly . . . a second area of interest, in close proximity, was Grenade Hill Forest – an ecologist's paradise. This had generated and grown over approximately ten years and took on the characteristics of a rainforest. Man did initially plant this area with vegetation that generates naturally in the rainforest but it was then left to grow and develop with little human influence or intervention. We wandered through and it was both a fascinating and educational experience. It also underlined how we as humans have damaged – even destroyed – God's original perfect world by our greed and our increasing demands for advancing technology

Was I finally growing up? I had always been one

BAJAN AFFAIR

of those people who rushed from pillar to post in museums, art galleries and the like to 'get it over with' quickly. I very rarely stopped to read the descriptive notices alongside the artefacts or exhibitions. Today, however, I found to my surprise that I had an interest in ecology. I read every single plaque and was even impressed. Now I felt I wanted to join the 'tree hugging' brigade campaigning to save the forests of the world.

Forgive me for becoming more serious (I keep doing this; it's this mix of magic and pathos that keeps tripping me up), but this taste of ecology captured my mind, imagination and heart. There are many natural healing properties found in rainforest vegetation. Due to global deforestation, we have already lost the chance to find cures for diseases such as AIDS, cancer and heart disease, to name but a few. From over one thousand natural plant remedies – derivatives of many already used in conventional medicine – only eighteen now survive.

God gave us a perfect world with perfect ecological properties and man has destroyed much of this. I had always wondered why God made wasps – nasty, stinging little winged beasties. Today I found the answer. In recent years a parasite had destroyed vast amounts of crops in the Caribbean. Many chemical pesticides were used to no avail. With little else to try, man turned to ecology for a tentative answer. It was found (do not ask me how) that wasp venom mixed with other natural derivatives, eliminated these parasites before the parasites destroyed much of the island's economy. What an answer to my question!!

As we wandered around, one particular plaque really aroused emotion in me. Allow me to tell you a story of a Red Indian Chief in communication with the early white settlers of America.

The Governor General asked Chief Seattle (obviously after the white man's scalp-taking massacre of women and children!) if he would sell some of 'his' land to the settlers. The gist of Chief Seattle's response was that land and air can't be bought. The land we walk on, the air we breathe, belongs to nature and no human value can be placed on this. He asked that the beasts of the land be treated with the respect one man should have for another:

'I am but a savage, but these buffalo are my brothers and sisters. We kill each one only because of our need to eat to survive. Teach your children this and may it spread to generations to come, the importance of my message.'

No doubt the Governor General concurred to this agreement and history then tells of man's greed and treachery as the buffalo were destroyed to make room for settlers' towns. I only pray that Chief Seattle, the savage (as he called himself), did not see this. I hope he died at peace believing in the honesty and integrity of the white man and that his message would be taken to the heart of these 'more civilised' beings.

A last and very quick quote of the same era was from another Red Indian Chief. 'Only the gods are greater than the forests. Those who destroy them are fools and must pay the price.' Was this wise 'savage' able to look into the future? Look at the abuse that has ensued during the past centuries. Our potential Garden of Eden, lost forever by callous man and his impatient need for advancing technology.

Here endeth the lesson from Pastor Pearce but these sentiments touched me deeply and I felt a need to pass on my views.

The drive back, in brilliant sunshine, from the wild and rugged east coast to the more tranquil west was fascinating. What a comparison of landscape and the characteristics of the raging Atlantic sea versus the softer, calmer Caribbean waters where our hotel was situated.

On our way 'home' we stopped at what appeared to be quite an exclusive hostelry. It particularly appealed as it was set high on the cliffs and the views from this vantage point were spectacular. We realised the food might be expensive because of its location but, had a need to satisfy our rumbling stomachs. We had not, however, appreciated just how expensive the food was until we had ordered drinks and were handed the menus!

Too embarrassed to merely finish our drinks and leave, we scanned the menu for the cheapest options. We ordered something akin to a shared salad and garlic bread. The waitress did not look very impressed – that is, she must have presumed we would not leave her much in the way of a gratuity. Her sullenness was compounded by the fact that we sat there, spinning out our meagre meal and drinks, for more than an hour because a rainstorm had descended upon the area and was powering up into ferocious crescendo. After the experience of the day before, we were reluctant to get back into the mini-moke until it had passed!

We found it quite amusing (sadists!) to watch the sun worshippers, below on the beach, running for cover. We witnessed attempts to protect books, newspapers and previously dry clothing as the rain cascaded from the heavens, and watched items being blown away in the powerful wind or soaked in rivulets of water.

During this period, I went in search of the 'ladies'. On returning, I found RT locked in conspiratorial huddle with a 6'2" muscular Bajan smelling overwhelmingly of ganja. The conspiratorial scenario came from the stranger. RT looked completely befuddled and confused! He was highlighting his deafness and inability to decipher the other's speech. As I approached, I could sense RT's relief. He asked his new 'friend' to explain himself to me. Immediately the man 'dehuddled' and became rather flustered. He seemed suddenly lost for words as he communicated with me but came up with something to the effect of 'were we lost and needing directions?' In retrospect, I am not quite sure what this was all about. Was he trying to sell ganja to RT? Was he gay and propositioning him? Had he thought RT was a pimp but, having seen me, written me off as too old and wrinkly – not the delectable, young, lithe-bodied Bajan lady he'd hoped for? Evidently this potential conspiracy was a man-to-man scenario and not for my ears. It remains one of life's eternal mysteries (unless RT knows differently!).

The rain disappeared as quickly as it had come. The min-moke now dry, we ambled along back to the hotel. However, en route, we did make a slightly unplanned detour and ended up in the 5 o'clock Bridgetown rush hour! Yes, even in Paradise there is traffic chaos as workers make their way home at the close of each day. We eventually reached our destination and, despite the delay, agreed it had been another wonderful day.

We felt a little sad to be bidding farewell to our faithful mini-moke as we deposited its keys at reception, feeling that our wings had been a little clipped. But we had not, as yet, experienced travel

Pauline Pearce

on the 'reggae buses' – a tale for another day most certainly.

BAJAN AFFAIR

Wednesday, 28th January

We decided Wednesday would be our rest day after surrendering our mini-moke the night before. We were both feeling relaxed and reaping the benefits of the holiday. Were we turning into beach bums? I didn't really care; it felt out of character for us, yet so . . . *good*.

We met our first four-legged beach bum today: a surfing dog.

This morning the waves were not lapping on the shore gently but roaring majestically with mountainous force. A tiny terrier was running along the edge of the water, eyes turned towards the oncoming waves. With impeccable timing, he waited for the most ferocious breaker and then launched himself into the water to ride the crest of the wave in a similar way to a surfer. He continued this as the wave died away, still frantically running in the shallow water, waiting for the next gigantic breaker. I felt exhausted merely watching him. I might add I did not emulate his surfing technique. I spent the morning reading, sunning myself with the occasional dip in the (by now, calmer) sea to cool down. The only 'stress' came from applying sunscreen.

Later, feeling suitably fried (yet too chilled out to worry about the damaging rays of the sun) we returned to the hotel for lunch. Little activity, combined with too much sun and too large a breakfast, culminated in a certain loss of appetite. However, being on holiday and allowing myself some lenience in respect of healthy eating, I was able to eat two copious pieces of gateaux and several portions of ice cream. Healthy eating was for home, not holidays. My conscience did not prick me in the least for this gluttonous behaviour.

The afternoon consisted of a snooze on the sun bed, allowing my lunch to digest, and then a quick dip in the turquoise waters to burn off the excess calories. RT and I then decided to walk along the beach to Speightstown in search of the 'chattel houses', which we were informed sold typical local souvenirs. Some were quite exquisite, as recognised by their price tag; others cheaper, cheerful and colourful – perhaps classified as Bajan 'tat' – but definitely recognisable as emanating from the Caribbean. It felt so relaxing, despite the effort of walking, wading through the crystal-clear shallows of the calm sea. I annoyed RT by 'snapping' (camera-wise) manically at anything and everything remotely interesting.

Our journey took us past the infamous Sandy Lane Hotel, which someone in authority had told me was the most expensive hotel, not only in the Caribbean, but also the world! A guest in our hotel had already spotted George Hamilton and Michael Winner in the vicinity. It certainly looked extremely luxurious from my vantage point. I noticed a large number of security guards patrolling the perimeter. Supposedly, this was to keep the riff raff (such as

BAJAN AFFAIR

RT and myself) out but it also gave the impression of a highly luxurious prison from which guests had no escape!

Would I really enjoy being wealthy enough to reside here? I would imagine the only parts of Barbados many of the guests accessed were that of the hotel, the gardens and the immediate sea frontage. Would they have experienced the amazing sense and feel of the island and inhabitants that we were so fortunate to access? With money, privilege and fame, perhaps reality of life is lost. I think my preferred choice would be living in the here and now, in the 'real' – if not so pampered – world.

We were soon approaching Speightstown. RT, kind man that he is, had been carrying a rucksack containing our possessions – money, clothing, sandals and so on. The Bajans are very polite and respectful people; beach wear is strictly for the beach and one is expected to cover up bikinis and swimming trunks in other public settings.

Hence, we observed the unwritten regulations and covered our 'bits' with shorts and T-shirts. RT had been carrying my flip-flops (borrowed from Beth – minus her permission) secured to the outside of the rucksack. Actually, I do not think in this scenario 'secured' is the correct word. I soon realised we had lost one of the two en route. This culminated in me walking painfully through the town to the shopping mall with one shoe on and one bare foot – most embarrassing!

A sign posted on entering the mall said 'No smoking. No loitering. No bare backs'. Would I be breaking this regulation by entering with one naked foot? I slunk in and dived into the nearest shop that might sell the ubiquitous 'flip flop'. Yes, they did sell them but at an astronomical price of £15! Unbelievable! The reason for this extortion, I discovered, was that they were imported items and, as such, were far more expensive than locally manufactured goods.

I proceeded, with great embarrassment, to limp out with my shamefully naked foot and into another possible 'flip flop' outlet. Praise be! I found an island-manufactured sandal for the UK equivalent of £3 and left the shop in higher spirits. However, daughter would now know of her mother's dastardly deed of borrowing sandals, minus permission, as on the new flip flops was emblazoned 'Barbados'. Beth and I have had many an argument based around her surreptitiously borrowing my clothes or shoes without my permission or knowledge. How do I explain this to her now, considering her original flip flops were bought at an extortionate price purely because they had a Miss Selfridge logo on them? The adage 'Hell holds no wrath more than a woman's scorn' seemed apt, if the words 'scornful woman' were replaced with 'stroppy teenager'. Still, this was a problem to be met when she returned from university and not one that was

BAJAN AFFAIR

going to blight my holiday.

We finally found the chattel village and bought (my guilt kicking in) some perhaps more expensive gifts for Beth than I would have usually purchased, including a second Rastafarian hat (I had decided to keep the first one for myself – perfect for keeping ears warm whilst putting out washing on a blustery Spring day!) Looking at Beth's hat later at the hotel, I wondered whether she would wear it in the wilds of campus at Aberystwyth University – warm, yes; colourful, yes; but *trendy*? Your guess is as good as mine. I still did not have a gift for my 87-year-old mother and remained convinced that it really could be taken for a tea cosy. I'm sure mum wouldn't know the difference! I could even be on to something big back in the UK – importing these unusual hats, modifying to fit purpose and then selling on at twice the amount of original cost. I might even be able to give up the 'day job' – not to mention all the tax-deductible trips back to Barbados to meet with my suppliers!

I think the sun was most certainly addling the brain. Still, it was a nice, if ridiculous, idea. Maybe needs a little more thinking through. And I must, most certainly, find another gift for lovely nanna.

I interrupt here, with a point of great educational value regarding the terminology 'chattel house', for those of you to whom this is a mystery. These original dwellings formerly rested on a brick base. When the residents tired of living in a particular area, the house could be loaded onto a large truck and moved to a different location. In theory this sounds superb and I wish we had a similar housing strategy in the UK. In reality, this was *old* Barbados. In contrast, these particular chattel houses were purpose-built for tourists and had fixed foundations. Yet I still like the sound of the original concept and even believe, in certain parts of the island, this tradition is still carried on.

Educational point made, we move on.

RT (now possessing a lighter wallet and a heavier rucksack) and I made our way back to the hotel, mission accomplished. Unbelievably, three quarters of the way into our walk, we found the missing sandal. We had thought it long lost and swept far out to sea. What a relief. I can now replace the borrowed items in daughter's cupboard – both intact and undamaged. Will I tell her the missing flip-flop story? Possibly not! The positive side to this is that I now possess my very own (more comfortable) sandals and will never need to borrow hers again. Plus, I now have yet another souvenir from our holiday, with a story attached. The day had proved remarkably kind to this most deceptive and hypocritical of mothers.

However, this incident has highlighted another potential area of conflict between Beth and me. I have also borrowed (again, minus permission) one of her bikinis and have had several photos taken wearing it. How do I handle that deception when

BAJAN AFFAIR

she thumbs her way through our holiday snaps? From here on in, I think – and have learnt from the flip-flop scenario – that honesty is always the best policy. As the saying goes, 'be warned. Your sins will find you out.' Most apt!

A final postscript before I end this day. On our return, I noticed a hotel employee running along the corridor close to our bedroom and disappearing through a door marked 'Fire Exit'. Was there a problem? I say this because most Bajans do not 'do' fast; they do not run, they amble; they chill. He was, however, smiling at us as he ran, showing off a set of glistening white teeth. This made me feel more reassured but I did briefly have a second most unkindly thought. Was he smiling at the prospect of many demanding hotel guests going up in flames? I dismissed this ungenerous interpretation moments later. Perhaps he was training for an athletic competition or something of that ilk and the running down (and presumably up) steps scenario was to improve muscular and cardiovascular strength!

These daily ramblings of mine, although enjoyable, are also tiring in the slower-paced Bajan setting. I will put pen and paper down at this point and bid a Goodnight and God bless to my much beloved island in the sun.

Pauline Pearce

<u>Thursday, 29th January</u>

I really impressed myself with a sudden burst of energy this morning. This might have been my conscience pricking me, due to gorging on copious thick pancakes with lashings of maple syrup at breakfast. I can also feel my girth expanding as each day progresses.

I knew our plans for later that day were mainly sedentary (I will explain our programme later) and guilt at my earlier gluttony drove me to exercise. This can often be quite irksome at home but exercise on a tropical beach and in crystal-clear waters is actually quite enjoyable.

I began my activity in the sea. This entailed fifty breaststrokes to the left, of base point and then fifty to the right. I was not even out of breath at this exertion. Amazing! Encouraged by this, I turned to aerobic weight-bearing exercise. When one reaches my grand old age, susceptibility to osteoporosis has to be born in mind – well, in my mind anyway. I cannot cope with further bits of my body malfunctioning, becoming damaged or falling off! With this in mind, power walking combined with running along the beach seemed appropriate. I power-walked for fifty steps and then ran for fifty steps for approximately twenty minutes. Good going, I thought, for an old girl. The release of endorphins invigorated me, kicking in the 'feel-good' factor.

BAJAN AFFAIR

I do have a thing about my age, don't I? Answers on a postcard as to how I combat this phobia, please. Communication from counsellors especially welcome.

Today we were collected by minibus at 11 am to go on a sea excursion departing from Bridgetown Harbour. Our exploration was to be below the surface of the sea. Our mode of transport was aboard a customised submarine. Our purpose, to view the coral and aquatic life below the Caribbean Sea. Yes, this was pure and blatant tourism, but also a wonderful experience not to be missed. Unfortunately, the minibus arrived very early at the port, which was most unusual for Bajan timing.

'There must be a reason', I thought to myself; and then I discovered the possible answer. On the waterfront was a most expensive gift shop and snack bar, both of which were air-conditioned and wonderfully cool. We potential deep-sea explorers, with an hour to wait before our Nemo Experience, were captive retail consumers. There was little shade on the quayside and the midday sun was blazing on our backs. Who in their right mind would choose to stay in this relentless heat when there were two beautifully cool outlets where refuge could be sought? Smart tactics by the leisure company or pure coincidence that our tender was delayed? I leave you to decide.

Pauline Pearce

I managed to steer clear of the gift shop (or should I say RT steered me away?) but the snack bar beckoned. I succumbed to an ice-cold fizzy drink and perhaps the most calorific ice cream I have ever had the delight to sample. In my favour, I was supporting the local economy by choosing an island made product in preference to an imported Walls or Nestlé concoction. Then came the guilt. Why did I succumb to suicidal dietary temptation? Had I not lost, in the lick of an ice cream, any potential benefit from my early morning exercise, especially as RT had merely sat on the balcony reading, having eaten less breakfast than me, with no interest in ice cream?! I had felt morally superior until that point. When God handed out willpower, he obviously allocated mine to some other fortunate mortal.

The tender taking us out to the 'sub' finally arrived. We sailed from the harbour and into deeper water. We waited in great anticipation for the sub to resurface. The previous passengers disembarked and stepped onto our tender whilst we reversed the operation. The sub, with copious portholes on either side, was well lit and less claustrophobic than I had imagined. We began our descent to deeper levels and eventually were only several feet from the seabed. We had entered a new dimension of oceanic exploration – a literal 'out of this world' experience below the Caribbean Sea; a kingdom of delicately coloured coral, of living, breathing anemone and plankton. Breathing beneath the water may seem a strange concept

BAJAN AFFAIR

but that is how it appeared as these amazing creations appeared to open and then close in rhythmic synchronisation with one another. Differing varieties of plankton waved gently as if stretching to the surface of the crystal-clear water; the sea itself changed in majestic colour and character from dark topaz to myriad shades of turquoise, dependant on whether the sun above was shining brightly or had been obscured partially or wholly by cloud.

The fish at these deeper levels were spectacular in range of species, size and colour. Many of them had names I had never heard before, let alone observed. Some – mainly the smaller fish – swam in large shoals, others in splendid isolation. I felt we were privileged to see these aquatic beauties in their natural habitat and not in purpose-built tanks in aquariums, garden centres or pet shops. We saw majestic electric rays; neon tetras in shades of fluorescent blue and yellow; black and white zebra fish; potentially dangerous piranha; anchovies. Up until then I had not even appreciated the fact that anchovies were a type of fish (yes, I admit to my gross, excuseless ignorance); I had eaten them on pizzas and thought they were of vegetable origin!

This was indeed a kingdom as magnificent as any of land origin and perhaps of greater beauty and sense of calm descended as we glided by as if unnoticed by life surrounding us on all sides of the noiseless sub – undoubtedly an intrusion but somehow not perceived as such. Life carried on in abundant variation, as indeed it would long past the time we would surface, in this kingdom that until now I had not even realised existed. All I can add to this is: 'wow'.

On board our mini-sub today was a large Canadian contingent of employees from the company that owned and ran this operation. I had thought it was a Bajan venture but apparently the Canadian company own several similar operations in different parts of the world. The Bajan outlet was out to impress and as I later discovered, our time spent in below water was of longer duration than the usual allocated half hour. I chatted to my immediate neighbour on the sub and discovered that he was, in fact, the company's chief executive. He was a most amiable man and answered many of my questions during our time together but, in retrospect, I wonder whether I overwhelmed him with my enthusiasm and excitement.

I was also cunningly hatching a plan, although it did not come to fruition. I impressed on him how much I enjoyed water-based excursions, many of which were run by this company on the island. I wondered whether he might offer RT and me a 'freebie' on a similar excursion. However, I obviously did not try hard enough or he read my thoughts and realised what an incorrigible, conniving woman I really was! Whatever the scenario, my hints fell on deaf ears and my plan

BAJAN AFFAIR

failed miserably.

There was an elderly, frail member of the party on board and I was told he was the president of the company. He reminded me of old Mr Grace from *Are You Being Served?*, a TV comedy series set in a department store, dating back to the 1960s and 70s (for those younger readers who may have no recollection of this). The similarities of the Canadian president and Mr Grace were that both had the staff 'kow-towing' to their every whim and a retinue of luscious young ladies in tow!

What an amazing 'Jacques Cousteau' visitation we had made to the underwater kingdom. My enthusiasm for this and indeed most of our time spent in Barbados was beginning to take its toll on RT. He compared me to a puppy dog in my boundless energy and enthusiasm for life. Although I did not like the analogy, I think that does describe something of how I felt. I did recognise a childlike quality deep within me – one I had never perhaps experienced before. I *did* feel like a strange conglomeration of adult and child and my behaviour, I know, reflected this. I felt, during our time here, the often self-conscious adult behaviour slipping away and I could be more open in what I did and said to new friends. I had a sense of the protective armour of adulthood being stripped away and being replaced, at the very core of my being, by the honesty and naivety of childhood. I somehow felt a new freedom to be 'me' with defences down; me 'au natural'. (Please forgive this newly divulged self-revelation – pure psychobabble I'm sure due to my psychotherapy 'roots'; or perhaps it's the effects of the sun once more).

At this point I will bring closure to another memorable page in my fast-growing diary. My 'affair' grows with the delights of each intense day and each new experience.
Goodnight, God bless, my treasure-filled island.

BAJAN AFFAIR

<u>Friday, 30th January</u>

We spent a rather lazy day mainly relaxing on the beach and with an amble along the silvery sands to Speightstown. This was mainly because we had booked an evening excursion to sample Bajan 'night life'. I did not for one moment expect our experience to be 'raw' Bajan, more a manufactured tourist event. However, we were promised, in the tour description, an authentic Caribbean banquet, copious amounts of alcohol and entertainment à la Barbados – calypso bands, stilt walkers, limbo dancers and fire-eaters. Yes, it did sound tourist manufactured and even somewhat 'naff' but it would hopefully be a different experience, whether of the positive or not-so positive kind.

I must admit RT was not keen to sample this event and I was taking him somewhat under duress. I knew my man though. After a few glasses of beer he would probably secretly enjoy the evening.

Back to the morning's activities. We had decided to wend our way slowly along the beach to the Chattel Village again near Speightstown. Within the village, we sought out an Internet bar run by a white English 'immigrant'. RT wanted to touch UK base and check his emails (can this man never relax?!), whilst my agenda was more to do with looking for souvenirs and sampling the finest cappuccino I had tasted so far on the island.

Pauline Pearce

We had visited this bar several times during our stay in Barbados and had become friendly with the owner and his wife. Today, nearing the end of our holiday, I asked how difficult had it been for a white European to set up and run a business here. Colin replied that if finances enabled you to buy a home outright, the Bajan Government would have little objection. Additionally, if you had employment skills that were needed in certain areas, that, too, would ease your passage.

I asked this in response to a local TV programme I had happened to see the previous night. The presenter had spoken of the rise of both HIV and alcohol abuse on the island and that they were actively recruiting counsellors. This led to my fantasy (or reality?) of finding work and a role for myself in Barbados. I really quizzed the poor man (much to RT's embarrassment) on the possibility of an English counsellor (me) working and living in this location. I plied him with questions, such as prices of housing, cost of living, and would both black and white Bajans accept an incomer? By now, as RT saw me stretching deeper into fantasy, he walked off and positioned himself in front of a computer monitor.

The reality of the situation sounded decidedly feasible for me but what of long-suffering RT? Jobs for 52-year-old, partially-deaf electrical engineers seemed unlikely. Would he possibly consider a change of career? Could he take early retirement, and would my salary support us both?

BAJAN AFFAIR

Would RT even want to be uprooted from the UK and make a new start in life?

I knew this sounded pure fantasy. I also knew living and working in Barbados would be quite different from holidaying here. Yet Colin (an ex-British Airways pilot) enthused about the move he had had the courage to make two years ago. He spoke of his home, situated on one of the highest points of the island, a vantage point with incredible views of the Caribbean. Colin was also an evangelical Christian, sharing the same belief and form of worship as RT and I back in the UK. His description of praise and worship in his local church was immensely moving. We had experienced a taste of this last Sunday in Paynes Bay Pentecostal Church and it had left me with feelings of new spiritual revival.

Could the fantasy of living and working on the island become a reality? I had set myself the task of researching this, looking at a timescale of four to five years. The weather, the pace of life and the people had made this a serious consideration.

If I look back over a number of years I have seen several friends of my own age succumb to the ravages of cancer – too many funerals attended, too many premature deaths. None of us knows what life holds for us and my thoughts in relation to this had changed recently. If you want to do something, whether it be travelling to far flung corners of the world, a change of job and routine or living in a different location, then do not procrastinate, do it in the here and now. As long as it does no harm to those around you – family or friends – and is financially viable, put plans into practice.

Hold fast to those dreams. Actively pursue them and do not be deterred. There's a whole wide world out there to taste and experience. Do not settle for second best. Aim high to attain your goals and one day those dreams could be your reality. Do not die with regret on your lips for chances not taken, for experiences unfulfilled. Live and love life to the full. You owe it to yourself.

I am sorry if my philosophising is rather overwhelming but I needed to pen these words for, perhaps, purely selfish reasons. If they were indelibly printed, in black and white, I would not forget the intensity of feeling on that special day and I may even follow my dreams.

Heavens above – this woman does jump from one topic to another as also the mood and wording leaps from daily descriptive narrative to something akin to philosophy (undoubtedly mine and perhaps not applicable to others). Again, apologies to the reader; but do cast your mind back to the intro – I did warn you of my eccentricity. 'Caveat emptor' – 'let the buyer beware'; be it property, cars – or, in this scenario, books!

To continue with Friday's events – after my words

BAJAN AFFAIR

of questionable wisdom – we returned to the hotel to shower and don our glad rags for the evening's entertainment – and what an evening that was!

We travelled by coach to the opposite side of the island and, joining up with perhaps a hundred other guests, were shepherded into a large open-air theatre with canopies strategically placed, in case of any sudden downpours. We sat with friends from our hotel at a long rectangular table, in full view of the various stages where the action would take place. RT was still a little undecided as to the wisdom of his choice in coming but after a couple of strong rum punches he looked somewhat happier.

Yes, it was definitely something for the tourists; but the whole operation was most professionally organised. The food was excellent, both in variety and abundance, and the alcohol flowed freely. RT thought he had died and gone to heaven (sorry if this sounds rather sacrilegious!). No sooner had he consumed his Beck's beer – his tipple of choice – than another immediately replaced it. The beer was ice-cold on arrival and quite often taken away half-full; once it had warmed up beyond optimal temperature, it was replaced with a fresh, icy bottle. This part of the experience was a little wasted on me, being teetotal, but I did drink copious fruit-based cocktails. Delicious!

I was conscious that as the evening – and the alcohol – progressed RT was becoming, shall I say, 'quite merry'. However, he was in good company as the other members of our party were steadily reaching levels of inebriation themselves. It is actually quite interesting, being both teetotal and working in the field of psychology, to watch individuals' behaviour change. The gradual inebriate is totally unaware of this – unless intoxication reaches the critical point of, for example, legs being unable to support body. I find, in Desmond Morris ilk, 'people-watching' fascinating. The alcohol imbiber thinks he is in full command of his faculties and is totally unaware that speech is beginning to slur and behaviour is becoming louder and more ridiculous. In this particular sense tonight, RT was unusually generous and had little objection to me buying not one but two Bajan music CDs from the gift shop. Normally, minus alcoholic joviality, it would have been far more difficult for me to accomplish my mission.

The cabaret began as we ate. What we saw and heard was superb. On several large screens the pictorial and spoken history of the island was told. The emphasis then changed to music and dance portraying the development of Bajan culture in both music and dance. The costumes worn by the dancers were incredible, particularly those representing Carnival time. Many of the dancers wore attire reminiscent of male peacocks in full and open plumage. How they moved, let alone danced, in such weighty costumes, I am at a loss to understand.

BAJAN AFFAIR

Stilt walkers standing a proud eight to ten feet also danced, and even performed acrobatic moves, such as somersaults and limbo under low poles. The compere informed us that stilt walking had a lengthy island history and that individuals go out to various
schools demonstrating their skill and encourage the training of youngsters to carry on this tradition. We listened to the traditional steel band repertoire and also to the more contemporary reggae epitomised and popularised by Bob Marley.

Before the finale we also watched the skills displayed by limbo dancers and fire-eaters. In the former, volunteers from the audience were prised from their seats and with loss of dignity invited to try their luck with the limbo pole. It is amazing what some people will attempt, once the alcohol level in the blood reaches a certain level. Needless to say, Miss Goody Two Shoes, in a totally sober state, dropped her serviette and literally hid under the table when the word 'volunteer' was announced.

I know I have told you, reader, on several occasions, that I do not imbibe the 'devil's juice' and perhaps that leads you to believe I am a rather boring, self-righteous character. Believe me – ask my family – I am far from that! I have merely discovered that I can find enjoyment and satisfaction in life without the need for alcohol. Happiness, in my opinion, comes from within and not from a bottle! (Am I preaching? Unintentionally, if this is the case).

The finale of the evening was again audience participation, but not in any threatening way. The reggae band played and we danced into the small hours beneath the light of a gently glowing moon, ending yet another wonderful day.

As we drove back to the hotel, the passengers on the bus were quite rowdy – not in any loutish sense but in high spirits after a well-enjoyed evening. I did wonder, though, how many of these noisy incumbents would be nursing a hangover the following day!

Good night, God bless, my special island. The days until we leave are sadly slipping away. How can I bear the thought of leaving you behind?

BAJAN AFFAIR

<u>Saturday, 31st January</u>

We rose early this morning (poor RT), as we were spending the day aboard a catamaran, and the minibus taking us to its mooring left at 8am.

As I drew back the bedroom curtains, horror upon horror, rain was lashing down and the wind was beginning to build. Not to be deterred, we boarded the bus but knew that if the weather conditions did improve our catamaran would, in reality, not sail. Even when we reached the jetty, the captain was undecided as to our departure. However, after thirty minutes or so, he made a definite decision that we would – in seaman-ship terminology – cast off.

Initially, the rain was still beating down but not as copiously as before. Rain on the catamaran is rather disastrous as almost none of the deck space is under cover. The only advantage is that whereas in the UK rain is usually accompanied by cool temperatures, in Barbados rain and warmth are usually bedfellows.

Shortly after leaving the port, the sun came out to greet us and the grey clouds began to disperse. However, the sea had much more of a swell than on previous days. This I loved, although many passengers were none-too-happy. I lay flat out on my beach towel on deck, gazing towards the heavens and feeling the swell beneath me. Perfect.

Pauline Pearce

The captain had introduced himself and the crew and he called them our 'Man Fridays' who were there to facilitate our enjoyment of the day, whatever that might be. The mind boggles!

Our Man Fridays plied us with morning snacks, soft drinks and coffee. Wonderful. No one was allowed any alcohol at that point, as the objective of the day was to swim from the boat with snorkels and masks and dive down to view the sea life below. Our main aim was hopefully to swim with the turtles. Alcohol would be offered after the first dive, as a safety precaution.

We, as divers, were told to choose a partner (or 'buddy') and to remain close and alert to any potential danger they might be in. Again, a safety procedure: 'you watch my back and I'll watch yours'.

My chosen buddy was Bobby. He was a very amiable man and perhaps twenty to twenty-five years my senior. The irony was that he looked after me, rather than it being a mutual arrangement, despite me being the junior buddy. Once I had removed my varifocal glasses, I could no longer recognise him amongst the group of divers. Was he safe? I had no idea. It was shamefully very much one-sided. I did shout his name as I surfaced on occasions and 'homed in', purely by following the vocal direction of his speech. He, on the other hand, had taken his

BAJAN AFFAIR

buddy role to heart and took great care of me. If Bobby had got into trouble I would have had absolutely no idea. If he, heaven forbid, had had some serious mishap I would have had to live with that on my conscience for the rest of my days. And what about the effect on 'Mrs Bobby', her children and grandchildren in reaction to my negligence and Bobby's possible serious injury or demise? That was something I did not care to contemplate further. I will draw a line under this matter now before my conscience and imagination turn me into a gibbering wreck!

At one point, I thought I had kicked another diver as I swam to the surface. However, looking below, I realised this entity was not of human origin but indeed a turtle. I (most embarrassingly, in retrospect) let out a spontaneous scream of delight. I think the other divers thought a shoal of piranha was attacking me or the like, until I shouted, 'turtles below, dozens of them!'

It was amazing watching the turtles in their natural environment, swimming so gracefully for such enormous creatures, and in such quantity. On land they appear lumbering, even ungainly giants, weighed down by their onerous shells. Yet under water it was a privilege and delight to watch their graceful and effortless movement. Some of them did surface. It enabled RT and other non-swimmers to view them, even if briefly.

However, to actually swim with and touch these

wonderful creatures was an incredible experience, etched forever in my memory. If only we had the reality of a time capsule that enabled us to travel thousands of miles across the world in the flash of a moment.

In this fantasy, I could imagine myself, A.M., counselling in the grey of winter in a Liverpool GP practice. Then in my lunch break I could be transported in minutes to the warmth of the Caribbean and the ultimate relaxation of swimming with my turtles. Would that Dr Who's tardis existed beyond TV fantasy! This, however, would have to be my own secret time capsule, accessible only to myself and possibly my nearest and dearest. Or would I even tell them? Exclusivity is the word. If time and space travel were available to all, perhaps my magical island would become over-populated and lose its inner heartbeat.

Saying my silent and sad goodbyes to the turtles, it was time to board the catamaran and set sail. Would I ever have the privilege to meet with them again? Even if this was a one and only experience, I will always have my memories to cherish.

The midday buffet prepared on board was delicious. The food was Caribbean - not a crisp or egg sandwich in sight! The majority of us ate on the open deck, balancing plates on our laps. However, with there being a moderate to strong wind (sorry if this sounds like a weather forecast),

BAJAN AFFAIR

lighter food items such as rice, peas or salad were whipped from plates and into the sea. Although I am certain there were no pollutant properties or the like, I did wonder whether they were of consumptive value for aquatic life. Do fish and other sea inhabitants need a daily quota of vitamin C in a similar way to those of human origin? Grossly unintelligent thoughts perhaps (no, definitely), but I have already explained my reversion, if not in body but in mind, to childhood. Pictures of mermaids enjoying a vitamin C-packed feast, courtesy of the passengers aboard the catamaran, came to mind. Pure fiction! Perhaps I would have more success penning children's literature.

Within an hour of finishing our meal, the catamaran weighed anchor and there was the opportunity for a second dive. This time the sea was extremely choppy and there was quite a long swim to the diving area – a sunken shipwreck. Only two of us entered the water. I think the sumptuous meal, combined with copious rum punches, had made the majority of my sailing companions, either too stupefied or 'chilled out' to contemplate the longer swim. The joys and advantages of being teetotal are many!

What a mistake, in my opinion, they had made. The second dive, to the wreck, was well worth the effort. Although there were no turtles here, the fish swimming around and in the wreck in Technicolor brilliance were more numerous than on our first dive.

Being unobserved (and perhaps unadvisedly, because of sea conditions and depth), I deflated my buoyancy aid to its limit. Although a wise safety precaution, it did lessen the speed at which I could swim and it also made diving more difficult. However, I survived to tell this tale.

We were called aboard as the anchor was raised for our sail back to Bridgetown. As I sign off for this day I feel that even though this excursion had been very expensive, it had been a worthwhile and incredible experience as we neared the end of our time in Barbados. I do realise just how many times I have used the expression 'experience' and wish I could find an alternative and suitable word. But experiences we did have, fresh each day and in abundance. Again, answers on a postcard gratefully accepted if any alternative words spring to mind. Or perhaps I should invest in a thesaurus!

The downside to this excursion will be receiving the credit card bill on our return to the UK. Before finally closing this day, there are some observations I would like to make:

1. On the dockside an Italian cruise ship had been impounded, so our Captain informed us, and the passengers had been offloaded. Apparently the cruise line owed 7.5 million dollars to the Bajan Port Authorities. How does that amount of money accrue? Possibly a prolonged period of unpaid

port fees mounting up, with extortionate interest rates on top of this figure? I really cannot imagine the scenario.

2. Speaking to a lady on the catamaran, she informed me that since losing her mother three years ago she had won £30,000 in quite a short period of time by entering various TV, radio and magazine competitions. While her mother was alive she had never been successful. I had always thought that such competitions were a big 'con'. Did Edna of Droitwich really exist? Now, perhaps all I need to do to be as successful as this lady is to 'bump off' my lovely mum. I also need to enter some of these competitions, as I have never attempted them in the past. So, 'Edna' is a real person, alive and kicking. It has been proven. The problem for me is that I love my old mum dearly and could not imagine wanting to harm her in any way! I think I am happy with my lot in life, although £30,000 is a lot of money to contemplate. I will most definitely *not* be engaging a hit man to carry out the dastardly deed. Yes, definitely happier poor and enjoying the company of my scrumptious Mum.

3. Since experiencing the rain of this morning and also the deluge when we hired the mini moke, I now understand why the policemen and women I have observed on the island have a provision on their belts for not only a truncheon but also an umbrella! *Non solem, sed etiam* (not only but also) – a Latin phrase learnt many years ago at school

– comes to mind.

4. We arrived at the hotel earlier than we had anticipated and made an instant decision (not many of these made in our by-now chilled out mood) to jump on a bus to Speightstown and make Internet contact with our daughter to encourage her through mid-term 'uni' exams. This was only a 10–15 minute journey, depending on how many times the bus stopped to drop off and pick up, but what a ride!

In Barbados there are two basic types of bus. The first are run by the Bajan authorities and the second, and most incredible, by individual private operators. All the buses are canary yellow and the charges identical. The journey, whether a mere mile up the road or to the furthest part of the island, costs I.5 Bajan dollars, which is less than 50p. On the outward journey we were the only white passengers. The bus was packed to capacity and beyond. The driver loaded as many prospective travellers as could possibly fit its interior, the reason being that the more passengers, the greater remuneration. Safety issues did not seem of any importance.

We heard our bus before we saw it. Music boomed from its high-powered sound system. 'Exact money please', we were told on boarding, as giving change is presumably too stressful. Passengers, seated or standing, gyrated to the rhythm of the reggae beat. It was fortunate that

BAJAN AFFAIR

we'd found seats, as what a turn of speed the bus had! The yellow-striped bus had what I suppose is termed go-faster spoilers. I have seen these in the UK but they are usually on – again my terminology – 'boy racer' cars. By these, I mean young 'macho' men out to impress their existing or prospective girlfriends, foolishly driving well over the speed limit.

Having completed our business at the Internet cafe, we boarded a similar bus. I had a real desire to travel all the way back to Bridgetown – its final destination – as I so wanted to prolong this unique experience. RT had to literally drag me off the bus, despite my protests, when we reached our point of disembarkation!

In Barbados, official bus stops are used by the state-run buses. These privately-owned buses stop anywhere, with an alarming screech of brakes, if a potential passenger waves a hand. To disembark one merely screams (to be heard over the music), 'my stop, please'.

This was great fun and an adventure in itself to a staid British traveller. I do not really feel this would work so well in safety-conscious UK.

5. My last 'P.S.' / addendum to this day was bizarre, yet enchanting. Leaving the room before dinner to borrow a stapler from Reception to fasten some of these diary notes together (I did not bring a notepad; most of this was initially

written on backs of menus, tour guides or pages ripped out of my address book), I found a note and a small flower partially tucked beneath the door. It read:

My dearest,
Our paths have crossed over the past two weeks. Your tan is coming along nicely, although I have seen your 'white bits' at the shower on the beach. I'm longing to speak to you. If your feelings are the same, meet me at 8pm tonight next to the shower.
Anxiously waiting,
Daniel.

Immediately retracing my steps, I pulled RT from the shower.

Was this meant for me? Daniel was a young man who worked on the beach for the hotel. I had approached him several days before to ask if he would take me out for a sail on the small catamaran belonging to the Tropical Escape. I had noticed him taking other guests out and it felt like a new activity I would enjoy to the 'n^{th}' degree. We did set a date for Sunday afternoon. I knew I would be away from the beach on the Saturday, and would under no circumstances miss the Sunday morning service at Paynes Bay Pentecostal Church.

Now: the note! Was it really for me – a middle-aged, 'white-ish' stick insect? There were so many

BAJAN AFFAIR

young and gorgeous-looking women, scantily clad in bikinis on the beach. Maybe Daniel was looking for a 'Mrs Robinson' experience with a more sexually experienced, older woman. In many ways I would like to think that. All 'girls' my age need some flattery as their bodies begin wrinkling and wearing, despite expensive moisturising creams, diets, exercise classes, beauty treatments and so on. I had only had my bikini line and legs waxed, plus two or three sun bed treatments. Unfortunately, I cannot afford a nose job, breast augmentation, face-lift, or botox.

I felt so sorry, though, for Daniel and for this luscious young lady – if the note was not intended for me. What an opportunity for two young lovers, and an 'old biddy' such as me had stood in the way! The only way I can feel better about the scenario is if I picture this not as a love story but perhaps sexual gratification and 'con' on Daniel's behalf. Who knows? I might have prevented this young lady from unwanted pregnancy or, even worse, some sexually transmitted disease. In that case, I have done some vulnerable young woman an amazingly good favour and deserve praise for the action taken.

I trust the reader will appreciate that I certainly did not keep the beach assignation nor, unfortunately, did I later have my sail on the catamaran. I actually laid low and did not venture onto the beach in the last few days without spies going ahead and 'casing the joint' for the ubiquitous

Daniel. Daniel also disappeared from Paynes Bay. Just a coincidence? I will never know, and perhaps it's just as well.

My heart felt quite heavy tonight. Our time in Barbados was suddenly slipping away at a faster rate, like sand trickling through fingers. Thoughts of returning home were gaining momentum. Yet there was still tomorrow and our much-anticipated visit to Paynes Bay Pentecostal church to come before our Bajan affair waned and eventually came to its conclusion.

I had thought I was finishing my daily account, but events of that evening inspired me to pick up my pen once more.

So . . . Welcome to the Party!

After a sumptuous evening meal, we took a stroll out into the balmy darkness of the night. All was peaceful and still, the tranquillity only disturbed by the occasional car, Bridgetown-bound. The stars twinkled in the clearest of skies above; the moon cast shadows on the pavement beneath our feet; our bodies were caressed by the warmth of a gentle breeze (I've got a little caught up in the romanticism of the occasion – apologies!).

The birds were now in sweet repose, hidden from the naked eye in the trees around us, only an occasional egret call disturbing the serenity of the scene. The tiniest of fruit bats had taken to the air.

BAJAN AFFAIR

We watched them in awe: dancers in the dark of the night, swooping then rising in perfect synchronisation to their musical accompaniment, the crickets (who chirped as if playing tiny castanets), and the distant sound of waves upon the shore.

A scene set for lovers, young or old. Love has no boundaries of age, race or creed. RT slipped his arm around my waist – a man not known for romantic gestures, as much as I know he loves me, with a mutuality of feeling from myself. Two middle-aged lovers, on our perfect Caribbean island.

We walked along, drinking in the atmosphere of the night. All was right with the world, in space and time. How could it not be? No cares or tribulations from home could penetrate or touch the feelings that we shared. This was our special, even sacred, moment. We were young and carefree again despite the ravages of time - our second chance over. A chance to be grasped that could so easily be missed; a chance that so few of us have the opportunity to take.

As we strolled, we changed direction and turned towards the shore . . . and then, the setting and the scene changed with immediacy and drama. Suddenly we heard the booming sound of reggae music. We'd been invited to a party – and what a party this was!

Pauline Pearce

We couldn't see our hosts at this point in time but, like in the story of the Pied Piper, we were led by the music until we reached our destination.

Dozens upon dozens of Bajans, peppered with a number of white guests, thronged the street. The volume of the music pumping out was intense beyond belief – booming, rhythmic reggae at its very best. As hard as I tried to resist, my body succumbed to the sound of its beat as if pulled by the strings of a puppeteer. It took on new shape and form – nothing forced or unnatural – total surrender, the movement overpowering me. I was a teenager again. The freedom from this was both exhilarating and exciting. I gyrated and danced into to the small hours of the night into morning.

This was raw Barbados at its best. The Barbados I now loved and that had caught me in its magical web. Black and white rubbed shoulders together in natural and rightful equality.

I had often felt uncomfortable in the realms of certain Bajan hotels. I found it difficult to accept that I was guest to be served and my black brother the one to serve.

Here, equality reigned – and it felt good. When islanders party, they know how to squeeze every last drop of enjoyment from the experience. The colourful clothes and hats, dreadlocks free and untamed – far removed from the often-stifling hotel regime. I had been very much aware of how the

BAJAN AFFAIR

black Bajans employed in the hospitality trade took great pride in their work and were more than willing to give their best. I had also witnessed some white guests abusing this and showing less respect than I felt was merited to their black brothers and sisters.

Tonight was different. The 'worthier-than-thou' white guests could stay cocooned in the confines of their five star hotels, whilst the indigenous populace partied and became true to themselves.

I felt a true sense of privilege that I was being welcomed to participate in this. One scene that particularly touched me was observing a couple of elderly white ladies gyrating to the beat with two young Bajan men – colour, creed and age were no barrier. Would that this be so, across nations and continents.

These young men were determined that their dancing partners would enjoy this party to the full, and they were succeeding. What wonderful memories these ladies would have to take home – memories to offer comfort and warmth in the bleakest days of the UK's interminable winter.

RT and I looked on, captivated by the scene into which we had unintentionally stumbled. We watched. We listened. We even danced. We immersed ourselves in this incredible atmosphere of happiness and freedom. There was never a sense for us of feeling threatened or excluded.

Rather, there was a sense of, 'welcome – come and join us in our festivity!'

All too soon, the middle-aged 'teenager' was feeling tired, from both the heat of the day and from the experience of the night. Bed was calling with the voice of Zebedee. Sleep was now the only option if we wanted the energy to experience Barbados afresh on the dawning of the coming day.

Thank you, sweet island. I take more from you than I could possibly give. Would that it were not so. Thank you for your unconditional generosity. Thank you from my heart.

BAJAN AFFAIR

<u>Sunday, 1st February</u>
<u>A.M</u>.

Our last full day on the island arrived, and with it the beginning of a new month. It felt difficult to accept that soon we would be flying thousands of miles away from our little bit of paradise in the Caribbean.

Our last full day, but one I was determined to pack to the limit with more Bajan experiences. Hence an extremely early rise to enable me to participate in my favourite UK hobby (but now Caribbean-style): horse riding. And to impress you with my enthusiasm – or insanity – this exercise was to be carried out before our final Sunday morning service at Paynes Bay Pentecostal Church!

How many incredible adventures can one individual experience in the space of fourteen days?

On the island of Barbados, there are neither limits nor regulations – only promises. As the sun sets on the eve of one day, the dawning of another brings with it an expectation of a moment or experience that will equal or surpass the one before.

There are no disappointments or false hopes. Barbados delivers with the sweet magic of its own. Such was today. Mr. Thompson, and elderly taxi driver, collected me from the hotel at 6.30a.m. An early start whilst on holiday, but when the word 'horse' enters the equation there are no sacrifices I would not make.

The late duty receptionist had rung our room the previous evening to enquire whether our early-morning call of 6.30a.m. had been correct. She also informed me that breakfast did not commence until 7.30a.m. This I had already ascertained, hence malnourished – save two bananas and a carton of fruit juice – Mr. Thompson and I set off towards the Caribbean International Equestrian Centre in the parish of St Andrews.

Mr. Thompson drove an extremely clean but battered black four-wheel drive. Despite its rust, bumps and bruises it was obviously a very dear possession, a car with a long and loving history. We drove sedately, at perhaps twenty miles an hour, inland towards our destination. The car bumped and shuddered as we hit the numerous potholes and gauges on route. The suspension (or lack of it) was more than compensated for by Mr. T's bright personality.

Mr. T had a beaming wide smile that lit up his face and accentuated the laughter lines around his beautiful brown eyes. The wide smile highlighted the fact that he had very few teeth, and those that were present glistened with precious gold.

I tried to initiate some conversation but it proved to

be quite difficult. Mr. T must have been at least (and I think I am being a little generous) seventy years old. Having few teeth and a very strong Creole accent, I found him extremely difficult to understand. He was also quite deaf, and I soon realised that he could understand little of what I was saying either. As he spoke, I nodded and 'hmmd' in what I considered to be the right places. I am sure that several times he may have asked me a direct question, and must have thought 'what a strange woman she is' when my response was as above – though I did vary the pitch of my 'humming' and 'ahhing' to add variety to the conversation.

We arrived at the equestrian centre. I think I had expected a grand establishment, as the name suggested, so was somewhat surprised when it consisted of a dozen dilapidated stables, barn with corrugated roof and an undulating, unfenced ménage. A Swedish lady, Elizabeth, who had come to the island after marrying an Afro-Caribbean over twenty years ago, owned the centre. She had been a dressage judge in her homeland, and now her main interest was in breeding horses for competitions. To subsidize this venture she had other horses that guests could ride on escorted treks.

Despite the appearance of the stabling, all Elizabeth's horses were well cared for. In the south facing stables, there were even large electric fans to ensure their occupants' comfort.

I was fortunate enough to ride out alone with my guide Garth on a well-muscled bay thoroughbred. In the early morning sun his coat glistened, accentuating the quality of his care.

Garth and I rode together for over two hours, initially through a verdant vegetated area before climbing high over rough terrain and then dropping down to the coast.

The views both from the high vantage points and the descent towards the sea were indescribably beautiful – God's creation in its finest splendor. Thankfully I had taken my camera, and snapped copiously as we rode. Yet I knew the quality of my frames would in no way reflect the full beauty before me.

Garth was an amazing young man. He was both an informative guide and a good companion. He shared a wealth of knowledge with me about each plant, bush and tree we passed by, and how many could be used in the form of natural medicine. He also gave me a far greater insight into life and culture on the island.

When I visit different countries, I have a real desire to learn about the area: its people, culture and religion. This, to me, is what the privilege of traveling abroad is all about.

It makes me sad to see so many tourists who

spend their time laying in the sun around the pool in their comfortable 'all inclusive' hotels. They measure their travel rating by the hotel facilities, the standard of their rooms and the quality of their food. They could be in Majorca or Mexico, yet have little desire to explore beyond the hotel perimeter. I understand that we are all unique in our choice of lifestyle and focus. God gave us choice from the day of our creation. However, it somehow saddens me when individuals limit themselves and miss out on opportunities to experience life in a richer way. This is but my opinion; I am sure many others may disagree.

Forgive me; I digress. We return to my expedition with Garth.

We finally reached the beach and stopped a while to let the wind cool our horses down. For some time, Garth and I were quiet as we absorbed the beauty of the scene. We were on the east coast of the island away from the more-populated west, where most of the hotels are situated. The beaches on this coast are more spectacular than the west. Here there are wide expanses of shimmering gold sand and very few people, the reason being that this is the Atlantic Ocean, so different from the calmer Caribbean waters of the west. The waves here crash majestically onto the shore, and the sea is more consistent in its deep emerald hue. The colour is only broken by the gigantic waves of white foam whipped up over the granite rock. No sane person would risk entering this powerful water, not even the bravest surfer.

I asked Garth whether the view lost appeal over time, as he rode this route so regularly. His answer was that each occasion he rides out he sees a picture according to the variance of the season, the sunlight and the sea conditions. In no way would this incredible sight lose appeal.

By now we had to shout to one another, as the wind blew stronger the closer we got to the sea. Garth signaled was I ready to ride on, and I made it known that I most certainly was. The horses by now were cooler and anticipating an increase of pace.

Garth and I held fast to the reins. The horses beneath us felt like coiled springs ready to pounce. I felt both excited and, perhaps, a little anxious. As we let the reins out slowly, the horses raced forwards and Garth and I galloped side by side in the shallow surf. I can honestly say I had never ridden at such speed. The fear left me and I wanted to protract this experience to its full extent, even beyond. The fifty-year-old woman took on the persona of a young child saying, 'I want more, more, more'.

All too soon our pace slowed, as we reached the point to turn off the beach and head back inland. I so wished that someone had been there to video our flight so I could relive these moments over and over on my return to the U.K. I will have to be

BAJAN AFFAIR

content with this being yet another experience to store in my mind's eye and trust that it will not dim over the months to come as the cold U.K. winter greets us on our return.

As we headed inland I sensed that Garth was comfortable with our new friendship, even though we had only met hours before. He was a very sincere, hard working and gentle young man. As yet he was not married, but did have a girlfriend. Soon they would be wed and his greatest desire was to have a family. His priority was to save enough money to look after his wife and children to the best of his ability.

Garth spoke of staying at his sister's house in Jamaica and giving her time to herself by looking after her new baby at night. He described how he would give the baby her bottle and, if she continued to cry, would hold her against his chest and rock her gently to sleep at the cost of his own slumber.

He obviously adored children. He said that if he was ever to earn a large sum of money his dream was to build children's home and look after those who were deprived of love and care in whatever circumstance. What an old and wise head on the shoulders of such a young man.

Garth also had an extremely strong work ethic. He was forced to leave school at the age of fifteen to help his widowed mother to support his brothers and sisters. He told me of the various jobs he had undertaken; sometimes menial, others hard, physical labour.

By the time his youngest brother was fifteen, Garth's subsequent siblings' income had brought more finance into the home. His brother was able to finish his studies, and even go to university.

This opportunity was something Garth had desired for himself, but time and circumstance were incompatible. I could tell that Garth was an intelligent young man and felt a real sadness for him. Yet he spoke with no bitterness or jealousy. It was just not to be for him, and he accepted the situation in that light.

Even though Garth and I had only been companions for a few hours I sensed a natural affinity between us, as we were mutually relaxed and open in our conversation. I felt blessed indeed to have had the opportunity of spending this time with him and trust that if RT and I are fortunate enough to return to Barbados, Garth and I can renew our friendship.

Mr T had, by now, returned to the stables to transport me back to the hotel. A very quick 'spit and polish' (as my old mum used to say) and an even quicker change of clothes; then RT and I set off for the morning church service, which, thankfully, was only a five minute walk away.

BAJAN AFFAIR

This was to be a bittersweet conclusion to our fourteen days on the island. The bitterness came from this being our last visit to Paynes Bay; the sweetness from the sense of the Holy Spirit being alive within those four walls and within those who worshipped there.

The service lasted almost three hours, but, as an evangelical Christian myself, it was three hours of Bajan Magic. How pristine, immaculate and colourful the clothes of the congregation were! The children especially, parading in their Sunday best; and the older ladies, in their splendid flower-bedecked straw hats. Presumably the reason for this is that no matter how little money they have, God deserves their very best attire. This was part of their act of worship. I could imagine that as soon as they returned home these splendid clothes would be stored carefully away in preservation for the following church service.

The rousing music added to the joyous atmosphere – an amalgamation of piano; keyboard; guitars; saxophone; cello; drums, tambourine and choir. Again, only the best and loudest praise to God. The clapping and cheering at the close of each worship song was praise indeed, directed to God on high – awesome communication between man and the Father.

As the minister, with such infectious enthusiasm, read the church notices for the coming week, I had a strong urge to sign up for Bible study, prayer meetings, evangelical mission . . . yet I knew this was my last visit to the church.

The minister must have spoken for well over an hour when he gave his address, but the time disappeared in the blink of an eye. Even RT (who at our home church impatiently times the sermon, unable to concentrate for longer than thirty minutes) sat transfixed. Yes, he of little patience did not consult his watch once!

Some 'touristy' ladies (looking perhaps for a novel holiday experience) found the courage to pass the portals of the church. Perhaps they did feel that the service was too long and protracted and that they were missing valuable time in the sun, as they left after the first hour. What delights they missed – even life-changing possibilities! They will never know, and sadly did not even care. (I should NOT be so judgmental. It goes against all my counselling principles).

In his sermon the minister portrayed many of an actor's abilities, but this was not an acting performance; it was sincere and from the heart. The Holy Spirit shone from his eyes and ordained the words that came from his lips. At times the message was shouted out so loudly (and this was with a microphone) that RT had to remove his hearing aid. At other times his voice would soften in a prayerful tone. He used his whole body as he spoke, his arms raised high to the heavens in praise and petition, followed by palms turned

BAJAN AFFAIR

upwards beckoning the Holy Spirit to come amongst us in the service. He did not raise himself high above us in a pulpit. He moved and walked among the worshippers. His pace quickened or slowed in tempo with his voice. Sometimes it seemed that he even danced when he spoke joyfully of his God and Saviour. Frequently he mopped his brow with a strategically-placed towel as beads of perspiration trickled down his face.

The minister made God's word come alive and his entire attitude of praise, prayer and teaching were infectious, leaving the congregation (well, certainly myself) feeling, 'I want more knowledge, more understanding of God's word, more compassion. Brother, reach out to your sister and touch her, not as a mere mortal but with the Holy Spirit that I see and believe is working within you.'

Nearing the end of the service a young man came forward with a personal request for prayer, as he was sitting an important examination the following day. The minister and two other senior church members laid hands upon him. They prayed for God's blessing and guidance to be with him as he sat that crucial examination paper.

I left that amazing service feeling sad that it would be our last opportunity to worship in Paynes Bay Church, and to praise and reach out to God in such a personal and freeing way. In my heart, though, I know that whether black or white, whether climate is warm and sunny or cold and bleak, we are all brothers and sisters in the eyes of the Lord. This much I have learnt over the past two weeks; a fact I already comprehended, but our time in Barbados brought that message into my own personal experience, making it even more real.

Yes, I do physically leave this Bajan church today, but I take a little of it away in my heart and soul. Each Sunday, after attending the morning service in my home church, I, remember my fellow Christians worshipping in Barbados as U.K. time reaches 2 pm. Somehow, I find great comfort in that and an even greater encouragement. Even time and space cannot separate believers from the love of God.

BAJAN AFFAIR

<u>Sunday, 1st February</u>
<u>P.M.</u>

I had wanted a final swim in the Caribbean before we jetted back to the UK the following day. The weather was still incredibly warm, despite (I was told) there being more white cumulous in the sky than is usual at this time of year. I had never appreciated how many different shades of blue exist in the sea, ranging from the pale aquamarine to the deeper colours of turquoise and darkest of blue. The sea looked so tempting that afternoon.

During our stay, the sea had been in many moods, which the locals said was unusual and related to bad weather in the USA. Some days the crystal water had lapped gently and rhythmically onto the silver sand, yet on others, such as today, there had been gargantuan breakers crashing onto the shore – impressive, powerful and majestic.

RT and I walked along the shore holding hands (I did tell you of the magic of Barbados. Would we do this at home after twenty-one years of marriage?). As we walked, dipping our toes into the remnants of the foaming waves, we watched the locals riding the crest of gigantic breakers on their surfboards. Brave people indeed but, for the not so competent, decidedly foolish.

I did manage the shortest of swims between these giants of the sea but in water no deeper than one metre, for fear of disappearing out into the blue yonder – swimming not as planned but sensibly, with respect for the power of the mighty sea.

Back on dry land we watched these magnificent breakers and the poise and skill of the young surfers as they rode their boards. This, in many ways, compensated for my brief swim.

We still had the next morning before we bid our sad farewell to the beach at Paynes Bay. We were due to leave the hotel at 2pm to begin our long journey back to the UK and the cold, grey winter. I felt sadness at leaving this beautiful island and its inhabitants. I could feel tears pricking my eyes. To carry on writing on that theme is too difficult for me to contemplate. I want this diary to reflect my joy and not my sadness.

Perhaps, after arriving back in the UK and a period of acclimatisation to the cold; the damp; the return to work; the blandness of life in comparison to that on the island; I would look again at my script and amend, punctuate, check grammar and spelling. But this penultimate afternoon and evening I would continue to live the dream . . . enough! (Through a veil of tears and a handful of soggy paper tissues!)

BAJAN AFFAIR

<u>Monday, 2nd February</u>

We came finally to the dreaded day of departure. The hours and then the minutes soon ticked rapidly away as the time came to board our silver-winged bird to whisk us away from our home of the last fourteen days.

I had never been anywhere quite like Barbados before and, please God, we would return. One can fantasise whilst on holiday in the sunshine, relaxing away from work and the problems of home, that to live in that location would be idyllic. I had often wondered, though: if one had the courage to make such a dramatic change of lifestyle, would the reality come anywhere near the dream?

I had experienced fleeting fantasies as this in the past. However, with Barbados the feelings were different. Yes, I could envisage living there, not merely lying in the sun and relaxing but working in a professional capacity – as a counsellor in a drug rehabilitation programme perhaps, or with young people in the area of HIV education and prevention. I knew my skills as a therapist could be put to good use in either of these two areas.

After only a few days of arriving in Barbados it felt different to anywhere I had ever visited or lived. I felt as if I had 'come home' – the feeling of fitting into the comfiest pair of slippers ever worn. I suppose it helped that language was no barrier, nor did it seem to matter whether one was black or white as long as you could communicate on a basis of equality.

What is it that makes me feel I want to return and end my days here?

Is it the people – their generosity of spirit, their sincerity and honesty? Is it the culture and the slower pace of life? I think perhaps it is a mixture of all these and a realisation that I am fifty years old and that I do not want to waste any precious moments of time ahead of me – again, the adage of life not being a dress rehearsal.

In this reflection, I think some of the comfort I also found and connected with was in my relationship with God mirrored all around me – both in the island and its people. I felt I could reach out and touch the Lord here in a way I hadn't experienced before. In that simple wooden church in Paynes Bay, I could hear God telling me: 'I need you here. I have work for you to do in my Name.'

What a revelation! Or could it be misconstrued (but well-meaning) fantasy grown from desire? It has only revealed itself to me as I pen these words. I will strive with all my heart to make it a reality, at whatever cost.

I know that for the next few years, with elderly dependent relatives in the UK, any change as immense as this would need to be put on hold.

BAJAN AFFAIR

However, I also realise that this could be my potential and much-desired future, and time will enable me to research into the practicalities of such a life-changing project. I intend to take on the properties of a tenacious terrier that will not release its hold until he achieves his aim.

I am strong. I am determined. This is my goal. This will be my 'mantra'.

To become a little less serious (now that this is outed from my system), I return to the here-and-now of several paragraphs earlier. Yet I feel a real peace now, having reflected on my life progression and projected future destiny.

Not wanting to lose a moment of the precious hours remaining, I had set my alarm for an early morning rise. RT, who had been slightly inebriated the previous evening, had agreed to join me for a pre-breakfast walk along the beach. (Please, dear reader, do not think for one moment that my husband is an alcoholic! I have several times referred to his over-indulgence in the past fourteen days. After all, he was on holiday and some slack had to be cut. The alcohol had been inclusive in the holiday terms and his indulgence in the locally-brewed Banks beer had been far less than that of other holiday acquaintances!)

RT, before he slipped into snoring mode (a further indication of over-imbibing) had suggested a 6am start. I, being alcohol free and more realistic, set the alarm for 6.45.

As the alarm rang, RT stretched over, eyes still closed, to bring cessation to the resounding din. He promptly turned over and went back to sleep. I jumped (well, maybe crawled) out of bed, had a quick wash, donned bikini and modesty-retaining shorts and t-shirt, and was ready to greet the day.

However, even minus-hearing aid (hubby does not sleep in this, you will appreciate) I must have disturbed RT, and he also crawled out of bed. He, too, scrambled into shorts and t-shirt, had a quick wash and met the same new day. Evidently, what had seemed a good idea at 11.45pm the night before after seven or eight bottles of Banks beer did not feel such a wonderful scenario in the reality of 'the morning after the night before.' Maybe conscience was pricking him after promises made that evening. Maybe his concern was that Daniel might already be down on the beach! Whatever, it felt right and supportive that we were, as a couple, able to bid some of our goodbyes together.

This last walk felt special – almost sacred. We were the only people on the beach and I could fantasise that RT and I were alone on our own uninhabited island. We hardly spoke but I sensed we both felt the same sadness at the prospect of jetting back to the UK.

Somehow, as we dipped our feet into the sea, the

BAJAN AFFAIR

crystal-clear water looked even more tempting as the sun shone upon it and gave more definition to the differing shades of blue and turquoise. The silver sand felt comforting beneath our bare feet and the picture was completed by palm trees as they swayed in the gentle morning breeze.

I felt a privilege to be in that place – to witness and experience the totality of the 'picture' before us. I emphasise 'picture' because I felt that what we saw and lived that morning would be indelibly etched in my heart and mind. I can somehow relive that scene even when thousands of miles away in the UK, and know with complete certainty that I will return, and that the picture will become reality again.

During my stay in Barbados I felt I had returned to a second childhood, mixed liberally with a dose of teenage vibrancy. I'd felt a freedom that I did not want to relinquish in order to return to the fifty-year-old adult that was me, in the here-and-now reality.

I was in self-reflective mood as we walked in the early morning sun. Even though we were homeward bound in a short number of hours, I still held some joy within my heart. We had made this journey and found our own little piece of paradise despite illness, stress at work and a close family death.

This was possibly the only holiday for which I had

not spent months in anticipation, leafing through brochures, reading the resort and hotel descriptions over and again. The holiday had seemingly arrived without the usual research or yearning. We were both too tired and stressed to anticipate how the reality might be.

It had been time out to relax and re-evaluate our future and how life could be, if we really wanted it to. It had brought a realisation that we needed more of this Bajan affair, to immerse ourselves deeper, formulating firm plans to return, definitely as a holiday destination and after that . . . who knows? There were many reasons for us wanting to revisit – many areas of the island yet to discover and (on a lighter note) not having had time to return to the nature reserve, to picture the indigenous green monkeys. That was excuse enough for me!

Later, as we walked, I really annoyed RT by singing a certain song over and over again, trying to change the lyrics to fit our situation – an example of the child within, trying to break loose, driving the adult RT to desperation. It was a song played regularly on the radio, maybe in the mid-1960s. I could not remember its exact title, though it might have been 'Coconut Airways'. It was about a Bajan man returning from the UK to Barbados to see his girlfriend. There's a pilot's voice heard over the music, welcoming passengers on board the flight. This flight was outward bound, whereas my version was returning to the UK. Here follows

BAJAN AFFAIR

my rendition – please try and think Bajan accent!:

>Oh, I'm leaving my Barbados,
>Oh, I'm going far back home,
>Oh, I'm going to see my mother,
>Back in Liverpool, UK

>Far away from sunshine . . . in the old Bridgetown,
>Back to UK winter, grey . . . the rain pours down,
>Flying home on Coconut Airways . . .
>But, one thing I . . . pr . . . ay . . .

>Call me back Barbados
>To blue and cloudless skies,
>Back on Coconut Airway,
>Next time I'll stay – I'll bide.

>Far away from UK . . . stresses and the strain,
>Far away from weather . . . cold and grey and rain,
>Perhaps, it's only daydreams,
>Perhaps, I'm pretty mad . . .

>But if I really want this,
>If I really try,
>My dream of living Bajan
>Will come true and be no lie . . .

....

Pauline Pearce

We ambled back to the hotel for our last breakfast. The 'last breakfast' scenario makes us sound like condemned men; perhaps in some way that is how we felt.

I sensed that RT wanted to quiet his zany singing wife for fear of meeting others taking their early morning constitutional. Eating food would definitely quell my lyrical attempts. Even I would be too embarrassed to sing with mouthfuls of croissant! Believe me, I was a well brought up child, and singing whilst eating was definitely not on the agenda.

After our final consumption of tropical home-grown delights, such as succulent watermelon, fresh pineapple and mango, we returned to a much busier beach where I managed a last swim.

Jet skiers were out and about beyond the potentially dangerous breakers. I watched with envy. Jet skies were for hire on the beach, but the price of this was well beyond our holiday budget. But amazingly, someone must have possessed extrasensory power and invaded my most private thoughts: I had the offer of a FREE ride with a handsome young Bajan!

Something strange here. Did young Bajan men have a 'thing' about the older, sexually more mature woman? Was it a 'mind' rather than a 'body' scenario? Was that one of the reasons I

BAJAN AFFAIR

wanted to return – something in some dark recess of my mind that, until then (pen in hand), I had been unaware of?

Was I subconsciously looking for a young Lothario, or was he subconsciously looking for a mother figure?

However, I reluctantly had to decline his offer. The main reason was that our holiday insurance did not extend to dangerous sports, which this was unfortunately classed as. Also, I am not sure how RT would have reacted to me being in the company of a young, muscular man oozing sexuality when the only oozing coming from RT was perspiration. But it had been flattering to receive the offer for whatever reason it may have been. The only other person I was aware of who had experienced a 'freebie' jet ski ride was a gorgeous, tanned, long-legged airhostess on holiday with her mother. The emphasis here was on young and beautiful: neither category realistically applied to me. Perhaps this young man was merely feeling sorry for me and I reminded him of his mum or, heaven forbid, his grandmother!

I now had to face the closing chapter to our time in Barbados. Having returned to the hotel, had a quick shower, packed the last items of clothing and handed over our key to reception, it really was 'goodbye Tropical Escape'. Fond farewells said, bear-like hugs exchanged and tears shed, we said our farewells to Bajan friends.

Sitting in the departure lounge of the airport, our plane had arrived to prepare for its quick turn around and our return to the cold and bleak UK winter. I could hardly bare to look at it. This was quite difficult, as it was the only plane on the tarmac and we were sitting facing an enormous glass window, which stretched from one end of the lounge to the other. No escape.

We had made some wonderful friends whilst here – both local and from the UK. We have incredible memories to warm our hearts, if not our bones, on our return. I have written copiously, snapped photos excessively and sampled, greedily, every sense, smell, perception and scene from this island.

I have used over and again excessive adjectives and adverbs to describe this island and its people – wonderful, incredible, unbelievable, amazing . . . Yet to use lesser descriptive words would not have conveyed my feelings in the way I would have desired or have been fitting.

There was little left to say, at this point, other than 'au revoir', and the meaning for me in every sense was: 'I will return'. My Bajan affair has come to a close . . . for now.

To continue writing on the flight, with thoughts of where we were headed and where we had come

BAJAN AFFAIR

from, would have been too painful.

So here ends my wonderful, magical, even mystery tour of Barbados.

        Amen brother. Amen.

Pauline Pearce

Tuesday, 3rd February

I awoke this morning to the sound of waves lapping gently upon the shore, drew back the curtains and stepped out onto the balcony. A little bird, similar to a sparrow, flew onto the railings and sang a melodious tune for my ears alone. He flew off as I stepped further out onto the tiles to view the crystal-blue swimming pools and the flower-bedecked bridge that linked one to another. Looking slightly beyond, I admired the almost transparent sea in its varying hues of turquoise and deep emerald green. Now I could not only hear the hushed sounds of the sea, but could also see the silver sand as it shimmered in the early morning sunshine .

And then . . . I woke from this most wonderful dream.

Yet in some *Alice in Wonderland* tale, Pauline was in the realms of reality. The reality of being in Barbados. No dream – living, breathing reality.

How could this possibly be? My loved one (Barbados) and I had said our tearful-yet-tender farewell last night as I prepared to board the plane. The affair had run its course; had come to its bitter-sweet conclusion.

Some explanation is required. I had not made my escape from the airport, nor secreted myself away on the baggage handler's truck. There had been,

BAJAN AFFAIR

however, an initial delay to our departure. This is something one so often comes to expect in these days of package holiday glut – too many planes flying; not enough airspace; planes missing allocated slots, and consequently waiting hours for another. The reasons run on.

We had eventually boarded the plane. The sadness of departure was diminishing and resignation, even desire, to return to the UK became the foremost aim. Perhaps a similar feeling to that of having a tooth extracted at the dentist: 'this is unpleasant but I just want it over and done with NOW!'

The captain apologised for the delay, and even explained that, as the wind was strong and blowing behind us, this would cut our journey from eight hours to six and a half. Good news. The cabin crew prepared us for takeoff in the usual monotonous mode. I know this is essential, but when you have flown many times you tend to switch off, or fantasise of volunteering to go through the necessary motions on their behalf. So ran the usual spiel: 'please ensure all hand luggage is stored in the overhead lockers; seats in an upright position with tables stored and seat belts securely fastened.'

Then the ritual sightings of emergency exits; floor illumination should main lights fail; usage of oxygen masks should they drop down (importance of fastening your own before securing accompanying infants); how to don and inflate life jackets with position of whistle and 'top-up' tube and the order not to inflate these in the cabin (in my imagination, hundreds of inflated Mr Blobbies unable to move); the removal of ladies' high heels before jumping onto the emergency chutes. Have I forgotten anything? Maybe I could manage a change of career.

By the way, has anyone ever located their life-saving vest? I have often looked and never been able to find mine. But face it, with a plane plummeting from twenty thousand feet at speed into the sea, would anyone really survive?! I honestly feel these life-saving vests, or 'veste sauvetage', are a figment of imagination – a mere ploy to help the traveller feel a little more comforted about the crash-into-sea scenario. Forgive me, cabin crew, if the life vests do exist; but why are they so difficult to locate (for me anyway)?

To continue . . .. The motorised truck pushed us forward and the captain began to rev the engines. This seemed to me, as a reasonably frequent air passenger, a little peculiar; but then I do tend to panic on planes. The pitch was 'high rev'–'low rev' in repeated sequence. Then followed a distinctly long period of 'no rev' and a strong smell of fuel, as the sound of the engines ceased altogether.

The captain made his second announcement:

BAJAN AFFAIR

'We seem to have a slight problem with one of the engines but nothing to alarm you' (me now terrified and ready to unbuckle seat belt and abandon ship – sorry, plane). 'The ground engineers are attending to the problem which unfortunately will entail a further slight delay in departure.'

Fair enough, though internal anxiety levels were rising. Pauline, the therapist, talking to herself: 'Breathe deeply. Think stress-free thoughts. Read your magazine!'

Then, the third announcement: 'I do apologise but due to airport safety procedures, passengers will need to disembark to allow the maintenance crew to carry out repair procedures. Unfortunately this will entail a *further* delay.'

Despite the announcement of imminent disembarkation, we sat on the tarmac for thirty minutes in what had now become a steamy, claustrophobic heat. The aircrew began handing around cups of ice-cold water to the perspiring and potentially mutinous passengers. It was, by then, 10pm.

In conversation with an airhostess, I asked the question that I feel was on many passengers' lips: 'Will we be delayed overnight?' She was very honest in her reply in that there was a strong possibility of this.

Eventually, a set of steps arrived and we began our slow disembarkation. RT and I and certain other individuals, preparing for the worst, removed our complimentary pillows and blankets from the plane.

Rumours in the departure lounge were running riot and tempers were getting heated. Passengers were tired, hot and hungry – a very bad combination. Many people had not eaten since breakfast. The catering facilities were running low, added to the fact that many passengers had little local currency left anyway and prices for coffee, sandwiches and the like were – as in most departure lounges around the world – extortionate, and of poor quality. It annoys me that passengers become captive prey, once checked through immigration. There is little or no choice other than to pay these ridiculous prices. Pay, starve or dehydrate! Yet few of us, if any, protest. It is all part of the air travel 'package' and expectation.

Rumours abounded and were:

1. Unless our delay was over four hours, we were not entitled to any complimentary food or drink.

2. One passenger reported that she had once experienced a twelve-hour delay and had to sleep nose to tail on any available floor space in the terminal.

3. Another passenger had endured a six-hour

delay with no food or drink available. On re-boarding the plane, the captain had to contact the UK company and seek permission to offer passengers a complimentary drink. This request was refused. (I must admit, I find that one difficult to believe.)

4. Differing passengers, who 'knew' and professed to be experienced air travellers, said the delay could be anything from two to twenty-two hours.

The fact was, nobody knew and the information delivered was sparse. The 'mutineers' grew in anger and size. To be honest, in some ironic way, it was quite exciting. I sometimes enjoy an adventure into the unknown.

Working as I do in mental health, I was observing a change in the passengers' psyche. From being the typical (is anyone typical?) self-contained Brits who, in general, only interact with family or friends, we were being drawn closer together in our common problem. There was a real sense of it being a 'them and us' scenario: 'them' being anyone connected with the travel company, and 'us' being the victims of the situation.
Bonding had begun, in a sense similar to us being sent over the wall to fight the enemy. People were communicating with complete strangers when in everyday life they might not even pass the time of day with them.

Eventually the rumours were quelled, and we

received realistic information from the tour operators. We were being bussed to hotels for an overnight stay on the island whilst the plane's remedial work was carried out.

Unfortunately, this process was lengthy and very tedious. We had to queue en masse to retrace our steps through immigration; queue to receive and fill in new immigration forms; queue to be given new boarding passes for our next outward-bound flight; queue for hotel allocation, and finally queue to be reunited with our luggage. Passengers were tired, hungry and frustrated. All most of us wanted to do was find a comfortable bed and crash out for the night.

Tomorrow was another day, whatever it might hold. Hopefully, we would eventually get home.

RT and I (and thankfully many of our friends) were bound for the Coconut Beach Hotel on the south coast of the island. We felt somewhat uneasy as we were told to leave our luggage on the pavement outside the airport. We were reassured it would follow us to our various destinations.

We boarded a flotilla of minibuses; I did wonder how these arrived so quickly in the circumstances. Did the airline know there was a problem before we boarded and the whole pre-flight scenario was merely to keep us calm whilst arrangements for accommodation and transport were made?

BAJAN AFFAIR

One of the rumours I did not mention before was that, on the outward journey, the plane had lost an engine and flew with only three out of the four. Scary! So, regarding our extra night's stay, was there some skulduggery in all this? Again, an unanswered question. However, if that *had* been the situation, thank the Lord we did not fly.

There were only ten of us on the minibus but, even amongst this group, speculation as to our destination abounded. Some, having claimed they had experienced a similar situation, stressed economy would be foremost on the airline's agenda and we had the delights of some cockroach-infested hotel before us. The other more optimistic view was that we were headed for first-class accommodation – perhaps a hotel in which the air crew encamped on their rests between flights. I hoped for the latter, but was up for adventure. Somehow, the desire to fly home had been overtaken by the novelty of this new scenario.

It was pitch black outside. We were driving in an area that RT and I had not explored. It felt somehow as if this magical island had another adventure waiting for us to experience. (I do occasionally have some strange thoughts whirling around the deep recesses of my mind – but then you probably know that by now). The feeling now was something close to being kidnapped, blindfolded (due to the all-encompassing darkness outside) and being taken to an unknown destination with little idea of what our fates would be. Perhaps I need to book an appointment with my own therapist!

Eventually we approached the hotel and began to get a flavour of what was to follow, as a security guard lifted the barrier to allow the bus to enter. No, this was not a high security holding area or a prison. The barrier was there to stop the 'riff raff' getting in, not the inmates getting out. My hopes were raised as well as the barrier, and it took a few moments for the reality of the situation to register. What a hotel!

After an ultra-quick registration, RT and I were shown to our room. It was a most enormous suite with luxuries to the point of obscenity. The space, furniture, fittings, remote-controlled curtains, bathroom with jacuzzi and all the 'little extras' of a fabulously expensive hotel were there, and more.

Although it was close to midnight, the kitchen staff provided us bedraggled travellers with a sumptuous buffet, and the alcoholic beverages ran freely until the small hours. It was an all-inclusive hotel, and we did not have to pay a single dollar for this gluttonous experience. The tour operator met the charge in totality. We were also able to have a number of free phone calls back to the UK to explain the circumstances to family, friends and, in our circumstances, work.

We had on arrival been told to enjoy our night and

BAJAN AFFAIR

would be informed at 10am next morning of the current situation of return flight. Having replenished ravenous, rumbling bellies, RT and I retired to our most amazing king-sized bed and slept like proverbial babies.

Goodnight, to this 'Magical, Mystery Tour' – as it was fast turning into ('MMT', to quote the Beatles – and it did feel a bit like I was on the 'wacky baccy'!). Thanks be, for the extension to our Bajan affair.

Pauline Pearce

<u>Tuesday 3rd February</u>

What a sumptuous breakfast, and what amazing architectural surroundings in which we sat to eat – a little different from the Parrot Café at the Tropical Paradise.

I felt like a child in a sweet shop as I chose from the delights displayed. The breakfast spread was totally overwhelming. Was it a gourmet or gluttonous experience? I must admit, although my plates (yes, plural!) were overflowing, I perhaps only ate half of their contents – to my shame, when I think of the world's starving billions. What could I exclude that I might have enjoyed?

A quick run-down of options to suit all: a copious choice of tropical fruit juices and exotic fruit; a similar range of cereals and yogurts; porridge, even in the heat of the Bajan climate (Bobby, who had been my diving buddy, told me it was a favourite of his and he had consumed three helpings); Danish pastries; croissants; muffins of all description; bagels; toast – both English and French ; a vast selection of jam and honey; smoked salmon and cold meats; hot food comprising eggs – boiled, scrambled, fried and omelettes; bacon; sausage; baked beans; mushrooms; potato hash; some spicy rice concoction; fish of every description; coffee served liberally by waiters who must have had eyes rotating at 360 degrees, as whenever your cup was almost empty they pounced and refilled it;

BAJAN AFFAIR

teas – breakfast speciality, Earl Grey, camomile, mint, ginger, strawberry and Echinacea, to name just a few.

Can you now understand my dilemma? May I remind you that this was a hotel, charging the equivalent of £400 per room, per night – far beyond the realms of personal cash flow?

Yet, despite this, there was something missing. 'What', you may ask?

The answer being: our recently made 'Bajan family' – Gregory, Pat, Charlene, and David – the staff at the Tropical Escape. They were not with us. These were some of our friends who had made our time in Barbados so special. Our Paynes Bay friends who were always open, warm, welcoming and smiling. The Tropical Escape might be unable to compete with the opulence of this accommodation, but it was the aforementioned people who had played such a large part in making our time in Barbados the experience it became.

The staff we met at Turtle Cove would not make similar contact with us. It was strictly: 'we are the staff to serve you. You are the guests to be served – no stepping over boundaries.'

I tried to make overtures in conversation but there was little response. It made me feel rather uncomfortable. The hotel *was* luxurious, beyond anything of personal experience; but, without the equality and friendship we had shared with the former staff, 'it was as nothing' – an apt (if slightly misquoted) biblical phrase. Even if financial means enabled us to access Turtle Cove as guests, my choice of hotel would still be Paynes Bay.

My belief is that money, and the trappings that can ensue, do not necessarily bring happiness. Happiness comes from within and from the way we live and perceive life on a daily basis.

However, whether it was the Tropical Escape or Turtle Cove, the accommodation was not of personal choice and my aim was to drain every last pleasurable remnant of unanticipated (and most welcome) extension to our stay.

The previous night we were told to meet at reception at 10am, when there would be an update on our situation. We duly met with the representative to be told the situation was under control and further news would be posted at 5pm. Several individuals exchanged aggressive words with the rep., but the majority of us were delighted at the prospect of spending the whole day in such opulent surroundings. I was ecstatic as the facilities at Turtle Bay were there for the taking, totally without charge. It did mean dipping into dirty washing to extract bikinis and t-shirts destined for the wash, yet what a small price to pay for this reward. I still had a supply of perfume I

BAJAN AFFAIR

could dab onto clothing to refresh them and disguise any sweaty smells (sorry, is this too much detail?!)

The passengers of flight MY6157 Manchester bound were a somewhat bedraggled group. I feel we were regarded with some disdain by the regular hotel guests, who had parted with exorbitant amounts of money to stay in such luxury, only to be invaded by an array of travellers on a freebie stay.

There was a strict dress code in the hotel, especially in the restaurant. Men were expected to wear ties, shirts and long trousers in the evening. Women somehow seem to be given far more fluidity in their dress, though I am quite sure if a bikini-clad female, covering her dignity merely with a sarong, sat down for her evening meal, she would be asked to don more appropriate clothing.

Many of the men were tie-less, and even more had exhausted their quota of shirts, including RT. We coped by rummaging through the dirty washing for the least smelly, least crumpled shirt. Again, it is amazing what an application of perfume can do and how a stack of heavy books (replacement iron) can perform miracles. Could I somehow incorporate that into life back home and save both time and money on the amount of clothes I wash? Now there's a thought!

Back to the morning of Tuesday, 3rd February. My aim was to enjoy the facilities and end the holiday on a high. The only problem was, could I fit everything into the allotted time?

I swam in each of the three pools; sat in the sumptuous Jacuzzi; sunbathed on the beach and swam in the warm waters, ate and drank copiously; sailed on the hotel catamaran, and spent far too much money on film for my camera from an extortionately priced on-site shop. I had used all films brought from the UK prior to our supposed departure, but now there were photo opportunities I could not afford to miss.

Perhaps the highlight of my experience at Turtle Cove was the aforementioned sail on the catamaran. A 'Rasta' employed by the hotel was in charge of water sports, and I had noticed him taking a guest out for a sail earlier. The catamaran was non-motorised and very different to the one from which we dived to see the turtles. It accommodated three or four people, was functional, safe (hopefully) and basic. The Rasta, who I later learnt was called Paul, was quite intimidating in appearance. He had long locks piled high on his head covered in an enormous stripy Rasta hat. His shape of head had overtones of Marge Simpson's 'beehive', but that was where any resemblance ceased. Paul also wore large reflective sunglasses through which his eyes were not visible. Initially, he was almost monosyllabic,

BAJAN AFFAIR

which I thought implied: 'don't communicate with me unless I speak first'!

I tried desperately to drag RT or one of our other companions from their sun beds to accompany me but without success. This was to be me without backup, but such was my desire for new experience that excitement overruled fear of being alone with this dubious-looking man.

Paul spoke in short commands to me – very much to the point of the exercise. He was 'hot' on safety issues, and I followed his instructions to the letter, no questions asked – total submission. This was quite unlike my usual babbling self. Part of this was fear of Paul and not daring to disobey; the other was that I had never sailed into deep waters on a small craft and I knew he spoke with a wisdom and knowledge I did not possess.

I donned lifejacket and crawled into position, sitting exactly as Paul directed. He pushed the craft into the sea before jumping aboard himself. He gave directions as to how I should move to the opposite side of the catamaran as we changed tack and the boom moved across. The fast moving boom was something that had worried me. I had visions of not being able to move quickly enough and either being knocked unconscious or dispatched overboard. Needless to say, I did not tell my companion this fear.

However, change of tack and subsequent position

of boom came about quite slowly (for the passenger), and I had plenty of time to move from one side to the other. Not so for well-practised Paul, who had to move like greased lightning once we had begun to change direction. What an experience! Something comparable to the highs I had experienced on Alton Towers rides with my daughter in days gone by.

As we moved further from the shore, the water became quite choppy. Some individuals might have felt a little insecure in this but, to me, it was pure exhilaration. I could not stop myself from laughing aloud, so raised were my endorphins! Paul must have assumed I was 'barking'. However, somewhere in this, communication barriers began breaking down. I told him how I loved being on the water in such conditions. When on a boat, be it large or small, the rougher the sea the more I enjoy the experience. This seemed to be Paul's excuse for us to travel further from the shore, into even rougher water and more powerful wind conditions. Then, after changing tack again, a little too quickly for my liking, he 'let rip'. Total exhilaration! Even that description seems too tame to depict our flight.

It did feel like flight as we skimmed over the water. No longer was it a boat; we were flying and soaring above the sea. Our speed increased to imperceptible knots and the catamaran took on a life of its own. The power of the sea in combination with the strong wind made the craft come alive. At times and at this speed, the catamaran was almost vertical. It felt almost at right angles to the water. As we flew across the bay, the warm sea washed over our bodies. I did have a fleeting thought: 'Do these boats often capsize?' I even voiced this to Paul. He gave no answer. Did this imply a possible 'Yes'? The rush of adrenaline to the brain and the total thrill of the ride, however, overrode any anxiety.

All tension, anxiety and responsibilities were cast aside as I lived in the excitement of the moment, freeing myself of every adult inhibition.

Paul and I were together on the catamaran for possibly an hour and as the pace of the boat eventually slowed, we engaged in conversation, for the first time. He had seen in amusement, the child in me emerge in my reaction to this thrilling experience. I felt confident enough to ask him some questions about being a Rastafarian. I voiced the option for him to say if I was asking something too close or personal. Paul began to let his defences (as I perceived them) down. He became very open – even smiled.

I had learned on the previous Sunday at the Pentecostal church that Rastafarianism was a cult. I had previously no concept of this and thought it was purely a way some of the younger Bajan males chose to dress. Now, being with Paul, I wanted (respectfully) to understand what beliefs a Rasta held. I began by telling him a little of my belief as a Christian. I said that at the core of my faith there was one God and by the resurrection of his Son Jesus, we, as believers, had the promise of eternal life.

Did Paul have a belief in one God, multiple gods or even a belief in the existence of God at all?

His reply was that he did believe in one god and that his name was Jaya (or was it Jehovah?). He was the God of life. This, as Paul expanded, seemed in some way similar to the Red Indian philosophy I had previously learnt about. The air we breathe, the land on which we tread and the oceans that divide us globally as nations represented the God of Life.

Rastas, at the core of their faith, hold that animals, fish, insects – indeed, anything that has life within – are their brothers. All living creatures and earthly features whether of human, animal or geographical origin, are to be held in great esteem and with respect. My friend said the core of his faith was simplicity and, in his words, 'doing good'. There was something utterly credible and simplistic in this, that had I been a person with no faith or searching for something to base my life and purpose around, I might have been drawn into the Rasta belief and way of living.

However, I did know, and Paul acknowledged this, that Rastas can smoke copious amounts of 'ganja'. Perhaps after 'using' this, life and its

BAJAN AFFAIR

mysteries can seem that simple. If the Rasta was transported back to the UK with its dismal climate, noise and pollution, and exposed to some of our daily stress levels, perhaps this philosophy might not stand the test!

As Paul had described the Rasta philosophy of simplicity in lifestyle, I asked how easy it was for him to work in an ultra-luxurious hotel where affluent folk resided. He answered that he just got on with the job he was paid for, kept his head down and said very little. This was the man I first met and judged without knowing the individual behind the 'mask'.

I felt, in some way, I had to excuse myself for being an outwardly affluent-looking guest. I told Paul the circumstances bringing us to the hotel and of not having the kind of money that would, in reality, fund such accommodation. From this and from what had preceded, Paul became (I sensed) my friend. We had broken down the communication barriers and were meeting in a place of equality and understanding.

The remainder of the day, although unique in terms of superficial pampering, did not compare to the catamaran experience including the privilege of befriending Paul.

RT and I ate exceedingly well – perhaps a little too indulgently – that fine day. Certain fellow travellers imbibed perhaps a little excessively. Yet my high came not from alcohol or ganja but from the unexpected gift of an extra day on my Caribbean island.

After our evening meal, RT and I danced slowly to the romantic strain of Stevie Wonder's music, played and sung by two resident artistes. As we danced under the clearest starlit sky, we could hear the gentle lapping of waves upon the shore. We felt sadness now, because we knew we were on borrowed time. Home and reality waited but, whilst we danced, they were still far enough away to lose their poignancy in the moments that we continued to live.

At 10pm, as requested, the passengers of flight MY6157 met at reception for a final update on departure. The proverbial sand in the egg timer had run its course. The end was just around the next corner.

BAJAN AFFAIR

Wednesday, 4th February

We left the hotel at 2.30am in preparation for a 5am flight to the UK. RT had slept for a number of hours in the bedroom, but I remained outside on the balcony, draining the very last sensations from Barbados – feeling the warmth of the night air on my bare arms; listening to the gentle sounds of the sea and the chorus of crickets beneath us; writing the last words of this diary. I could not waste any of these moments in sleep. Sleep was, if possible, for the flight. Sleep was definitely for the UK. Sleep was not for these final hours.

On the balcony at 1am, I felt like the only person alive in this idyllic world. But my seductive, tempting lover – Barbados – was fading away, as the hands on my watch moved closer to 2.30am. I could not stop time. I could do nothing to resist closure to my Bajan affair.

This was finality, and there would be no further chances.

This, too, was where I wanted to rest my pen and leave a part of myself – not, perhaps at Turtle Cove – but certainly in Barbados.

When I read this manuscript over in months or years to come, I knew I would want to recapture the magic that permeated my body and soul at that particular time. I did not want my last words to

Pauline Pearce

be about the frustration of the airport procedure or the details of sitting for eight uncomfortable hours on a plane, nor indeed the reality that awaited on arrival in the UK.

Now seemed the perfect time to bid a final adieu to my seductive island and to all the friends we had made.

As surely as the sun set in crimson glory on each day and rose in greeting on the next, there came with each dawning both the anticipated and the unexpected waiting to be lived in experience and imprinted in mind, memory and heart.

I know the words I have used to describe you, my island, have perhaps been insufficient to convey your true beauty; but, as I bid farewell, a part of you is etched eternally within my soul until I come to greet you again – the seducer and the lover reunited.

Our affair will continue. This is my promise. 'Til then, this must suffice.

God bless and au revoir.

BAJAN AFFAIR

Epilogue

(Dedicated to my friend and sailing companion – Paul)

Dear Paul,

As I bring closure to my work, I have a sense deep within that my words may fail to express the essence of Barbados; that I may not have described the feelings within my heart that touch me to the core of my being.

This is *not* about me or my pride in making my words look pleasing on paper. It is about the island – about its inner heartbeat and beauty not in a mere physical sense but in the beauty of its people also and their generosity of spirit.

The word that comes with ease to me is 'God' and His creation - His creation of Barbados.

Here, I have felt His Spirit within me and around me, caressing me as a lover; protecting me as a father: 'In the valley of death, I will feel no ill.'

God was the first and the great 'I Am' and all began with Him – be He the God of the Rasta or the Christian.

In my smallness of mind, I had thought there was but one creator – the God of Christianity, the 'three-in-one'. The God of my perception; Jesus, His Son who came to live as man and died to bare our sin and God the Holy Spirit – His presence unseen but walking alongside us, in the darkness and the light. God whose footprints tread upon the sand, who carries us upon His shoulders when we are in despair and need Him most.

Now my eyes and ears have less restriction, and I hear of the God of the Rasta. Now I sense He could be my God also. At first I did not understand but my friend, you have helped my eyes to open and broaden my perception.

How could I have been so blind? How could I have been so deaf? How could I box my God into something so small and say He is but the God of the Christian?

Thank you, my friend, for helping me find OUR God with deeper understanding – the Father who loves his children with a passion deep and wide; the Father who shows compassion to all who seek His face.

I know we may disagree on scripture great or small but one thing we both know is that God OUR Father made a perfect world when He created man and woman, and the beasts of land, of sea, of sky.

I realise this anew when I am at peace on this island – when I've time to rest and time to think,

BAJAN AFFAIR

away from all distraction.

My friend, Paul, you have been the one to help me understand that God is all around us. That our Father is in the depths of the ocean; on the green and verdant land; in the bluest skies of day and the darkest skies of night. He is the one who flung the stars into the heavens and made them twinkle and shine, like the rarest most precious of jewels.

He made the rain to refresh the barren land and the plants that grow thereon. He made the warm and gentle breezes and gave almighty strength to the winds that roar and rage. This was His work and on the island, I see this – my eyes open wide, my ears more attentive, my senses more acute.

I thank God for the beauty of this island, and I thank you, my friend, for new insight and new understanding as we stand shoulder-to-shoulder, brother and sister. Nothing can divide us from God's great love – neither land nor sea, race nor creed. We live in harmony with Him and all Creation, and it is good.

Pauline Pearce

www.ingramcontent.com/pod-product-compliance
Lightning Source LLC
Chambersburg PA
CBHW032125090426
42743CB00007B/474